MW01059254

Fertility *for Beginners*

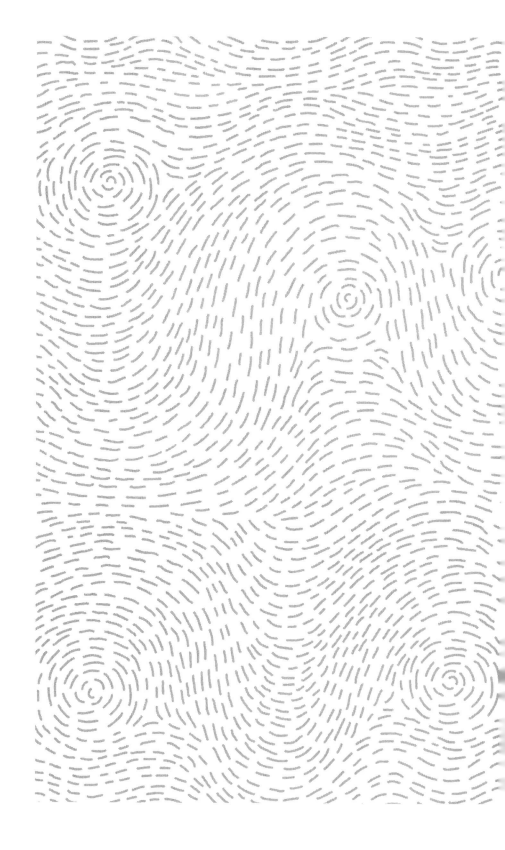

Fertility *for Beginners*

THE FERTILITY DIET AND HEALTH PLAN TO START MAXIMIZING YOUR FERTILITY

SHASTA PRESS

Copyright © 2013 by Shasta Press, Berkeley, California

No part of this publication may be reproduced, stored in a retrieval system or transmitted in any form or by any means, electronic, mechanical, photocopying, recording, scanning or otherwise, except as permitted under Section 107 or 108 of the 1976 United States Copyright Act, without the prior written permission of the publisher. Requests to the publisher for permission should be addressed to the Permissions Department, Shasta Press, 918 Parker St., Suite A-12, Berkeley, CA 94710.

Limit of Liability/Disclaimer of Warranty: The publisher and the author make no representations or warranties with respect to the accuracy or completeness of the contents of this work and specifically disclaim all warranties, including without limitation warranties of fitness for a particular purpose. No warranty may be created or extended by sales or promotional materials. The advice and strategies contained herein may not be suitable for every situation. This work is sold with the understanding that the publisher is not engaged in rendering medical, legal or other professional advice or services. If professional assistance is required, the services of a competent professional person should be sought. Neither the publisher nor the author shall be liable for damages arising herefrom. The fact that an individual, organization or website is referred to in this work as a citation and/or potential source of further information does not mean that the author or the publisher endorses the information the individual, organization or website may provide or recommendations they/it may make. Further, readers should be aware that Internet websites listed in this work may have changed or disappeared between when this work was written and when it is read.

For general information on our other products and services or to obtain technical support, please contact our Customer Care Department within the United States at (866) 744-2665, or outside the United States at (510) 253-0500.

Shasta Press publishes its books in a variety of electronic and print formats. Some content that appears in print may not be available in electronic books, and vice versa.

TRADEMARKS: Shasta Press and the Shasta Press logo are trademarks or registered trademarks of Callisto Media Inc. and/or its affiliates, in the United States and other countries, and may not be used without written permission. All other trademarks are the property of their respective owners. Shasta Press is not associated with any product or vendor mentioned in this book.

ISBN: Print 978-1-62315-307-6 | eBook 978-1-62315-339-7

Contents

Recipes

Introduction

Most couples assume that getting pregnant will be simple. After all, people have been doing it for thousands of years. But in fact, many couples experience infertility once they've decided to start a family. And trying to get pregnant when your body just won't cooperate is an exercise in frustration. Sometimes the reasons for infertility are medical, but much of the time, a few changes in your lifestyle—such as altering your diet and finding more time to relax—will take care of the infertility problems.

This book is designed for people who want to improve their fertility naturally. Here, you will explore your anatomy to develop an understanding of the physical signs of fertility. You will learn the most important changes to make to your lifestyle in order to enhance your fertility and how to achieve these changes. And you will discover the importance of the fertility diet as a natural way to optimize fertility.

Fertility for Beginners offers simple changes to the way you eat that may reduce or eliminate infertility. The fertility diet suggested in these pages is based on a study conducted by the Harvard School of Public Health, with the participation of more than eighteen thousand female nurses. The study, which began in 1989, looked at the effect the nurses' diets had on their fertility. It was part of a larger investigation, begun in 1976, that studied how diet, lifestyle, and social and biological factors affect the risk of diabetes, heart disease, and other chronic health conditions.

In this book we focus on the results of the smaller study of diet and fertility.

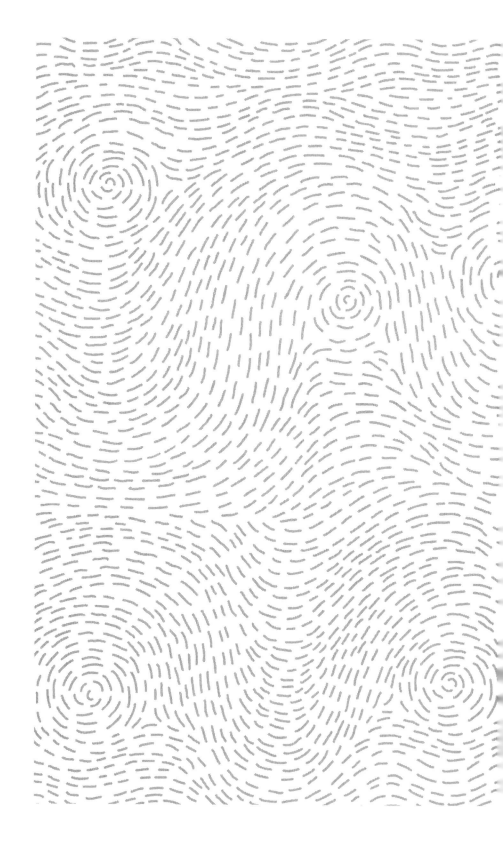

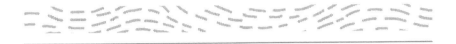

PART ONE

The Fertility Diet

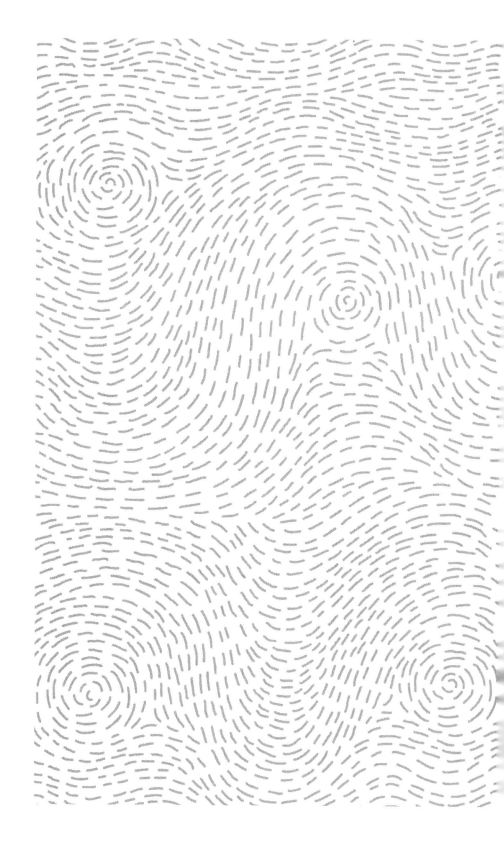

CHAPTER ONE

Understanding Fertility

Getting pregnant is something we take for granted, a biological process that is a built-in part of our mammalian selves. Women are taught from a very young age about their body's ability to become pregnant and frequently, how to prevent pregnancy. If you are reading this book, you probably have been trying to conceive, but it has not happened. You want to keep trying, so you are looking for ways to improve your chances of getting pregnant.

Many couples who have been unsuccessfully trying to conceive often look to assisted reproductive technologies (ARTs), such as drugs that increase egg production, or in vitro fertilization (IVF), which involves fertilizing a woman's egg outside of her womb for implantation later. In our always-in-a-hurry society, technology seems to many like the best path to reaching the goal of conception, pregnancy, and parenthood. In fact, the number of families seeking IVF has dramatically increased since it was first introduced in 1978.

Conception and birth are cause for celebration, no matter how the birth was achieved. Indeed, these advanced technologies are something of a miracle for families who have tried for years to conceive naturally. However, they are not perfect. They lead to a viable pregnancy about 25 percent of the time. ARTs can also be expensive and time-consuming, and have unpleasant side effects.

This book offers a more natural path to increasing fertility. It supports every woman who is attempting to become pregnant by looking at diet, nutrition, and lifestyle choices that will improve her chances. These natural choices also have a positive impact on couples who do choose to use ARTs to conceive. Let's begin with lifestyle.

FACTORS THAT AFFECT FERTILITY

Factors such as exercise, travel, weight, stress, age, and vaginal infections can all affect your fertility. Let's take a look at each one.

Exercise

Strenuous exercise can delay or even prevent ovulation. This is especially true of competitive athletes who have a very low ratio of body fat to total body weight. The studies done on athletes are somewhat inconclusive, however, as the researchers did not separate the negative impacts of stress, travel, and diet on these athletes.

Many athletes speak of the runner's high they experience when exercising vigorously. This feeling of euphoria is caused by the release of a flood of chemicals, called endorphins, in the brain. Endorphins increase the body's levels of prolactin, which a woman's body releases for the production of breast milk. An increase in prolactin may decrease the possibility of pregnancy. What is notable for our purposes is that exercise at the competitive level has a negative impact on fertility. But moderate exercise—one hour a day, three days a week—should become a part of your fertility lifestyle, if it is not already.

Travel

We may be quite accustomed to the idea of traveling from one time zone to another, even from one continent to another, in a matter of hours. Our bodies, however, are not so quick to adapt to modern travel and may find it stressful. While one woman may have no physical side effects from travel, another may experience a lot of change—from the timing of her menstrual cycle to her circadian rhythm (the twenty-four-hour rhythm of biological activity and rest that our bodies are attuned to every day). Some women stop menstruating or stop ovulating altogether when they travel. By noting travel on a fertility chart, we can see how travel is affecting our menstrual rhythm and how it may be impacting our wellness.

Weight

Sex hormones are fat soluble, and our body fat stores hormones such as estrogen. Fat also converts a hormone called androgen into a type of estrogen necessary for ovulation to occur. Our bodies must have enough fat in order to function properly for overall wellness, as well as for fertility. A woman should have at least 20 percent of her body weight as fat.

Underweight women and women with less than 20 percent body fat may not produce enough estrogen and other hormones to menstruate or ovulate. Overweight women and those with more than 20 percent body fat can produce too much estrogen and other hormones, which may prevent ovulation. There is some wiggle room built into these body fat numbers, often referred to as the body mass index (BMI). In general, you do not want your BMI to drop below 19 percent or rise above 25 percent body fat. Discuss any concerns about weight or irregular cycles with your health-care practitioner.

Stress

Psychological and physiological stress tends to delay ovulation. There are other ways that stress can negatively impact ovulation, as well. A busy life, one full of business and social obligations, can reduce the time you spend with your partner, and therefore the frequency of intercourse. And just the fact that you are not achieving pregnancy in any given cycle can cause stress.

The gland in the brain called the hypothalamus controls much of the reproductive system. It has the important job of linking the nervous system to the endocrine system—the cells, glands, and tissues that secrete hormones into the bloodstream via the pituitary gland. The pituitary gland is responsible for releasing follicle-stimulating hormone (FSH) and luteinizing hormone (LH). FSH and LH are needed for a woman's ovaries to release a mature egg. When stress impacts the hypothalamus, the release of these reproductive hormones from the pituitary gland is delayed, resulting in a longer menstrual cycle. If stress is severe, it can prevent ovulation from happening at all. (This is known as an anovulatory cycle.) By keeping track of your fertility signs, including any signs of stress on your cycle, you can identify when you are about to ovulate.

Age

There is no doubt that age is a factor in fertility. The physiological changes a woman experiences as she ages directly affects her fertility rates. The quality and quantity of cervical fluid begins to decline. The number of anovulatory cycles increases. The luteal phase, the postovulatory phase of your menstrual cycle, gets shorter.

Gloomier still are the numbers related to miscarriages. For women under the age of 30, about 10 percent of pregnancies end in miscarriage, while for women between 35 and 39, 18 percent end in miscarriage. For women between 40 and 44, about 34 percent of pregnancies supposedly end in miscarriage, but some statistics show a miscarriage rate for this group as high as 50 percent, most of which are not detected. The reason for the high percentage? As a woman ages, her eggs age right along with her. Her eggs have more abnormalities and produce unsustainable embryos.

Over and over again, the numbers show that the younger you are, the easier it is to become and remain pregnant. Peak fertility is a gift given to the young. Women under 25 have a 96 percent chance of conceiving within a year. As you might expect, numbers decline from there. But on the positive side, for all women between 35 and 44, 78 percent of them will statistically be able to get pregnant within a year. You read that right: three-quarters of all women ages 35 to 44 will be able to get pregnant within a year.

If you examine the statistics by month, however, they look dim. When a woman is under the age of 30, her chance of getting pregnant in any given cycle is just 20 percent. If she is over the age of 40, her chance of getting pregnant during any given cycle is just 5 percent.

How does the age of the male partner affect a couple's fertility? According to a study done in France to look at the effects of a man's age on his fertility, pregnancy rates fell 10 percent when a man reached the age of 35, and by 20 percent when he was 45, regardless of his female partner's age. Miscarriage rates, too, began to rise once men were in their mid-thirties. One in three couples experienced a miscarriage when the man was 45 or older.

We live in a world where reproductive technology enables a woman to freeze her eggs and actually defrost them at a later time, when she is ready to have children. (The technology to freeze sperm has existed since 1983.) You may harvest your eggs in your twenties, when they are healthiest, put them into cold storage, and retrieve them for fertilization and implantation. These technologies, however, are in their infancy, are very expensive, and are not yet widely available.

Although older women take longer to get pregnant, have higher-risk pregnancies, and experience more miscarriages, there are many steps they can take to improve their fertility. As you get older, lifestyle choices matter more. When you are in your early twenties, partying every weekend, not getting enough sleep, and eating a poor diet will probably not affect your ability to get pregnant. Once you pass your peak fertility years, though, lifestyle choices will have greater significance.

You can counteract the effects of aging on your fertility by making changes to your lifestyle and diet that will maximize your chances of getting pregnant.

Vaginal Infections

Almost every woman will, at some point in her life, experience a vaginal infection. From a fertility standpoint, about 15 percent of infertility cases can be traced to an infection. An infection may also cause pregnancy loss. Many of them, including sexually transmitted infections (STIs) are "silent," in that the body exhibits no observable symptoms. One infection that is often silent is chlamydia; more than half the time, a woman with chlamydia exhibits no symptoms. If the infection is undiagnosed, there is more than a 50 percent chance that it will develop into pelvic inflammatory disease (PID), a generic term for an infection of the uterus, fallopian tubes, or ovaries. PID can cause scarring of the fallopian tubes and increases the risk of infertility as well as an ectopic pregnancy.

Chlamydia can linger for months or years before it is discovered. A woman's symptoms may include unusual vaginal bleeding or discharge, pain in the abdomen, fever, painful urination, or the urge to urinate more frequently than usual. Men are vulnerable to this infection, too. They may have some discharge from the penis or feel a burning sensation when urinating. Whether they know it or not, between 5 and 10 percent of women and men carry the chlamydia bacteria, more than twice the level of a decade ago. Both partners must be treated with antibiotics if one is diagnosed with an infection.

Not all vaginal infections are STIs. A monogamous relationship does not protect you from all of them. Your infection may be caused by yeast cells, or you may become irritated by a chemical in a cream or spray, for example.

The symptoms of infection—if there are any—can mask what is going on with your cervical fluid. Once you are familiar with your own cervical fluid, any changes can be clearly spotted. (For detailed information on women's general and gynecological health, consult a good reference book, such as *Our Bodies, Ourselves: A New Edition for a New Era* by the Boston Women's Health Book Collective, published in 2005.) Symptoms of a vaginal infection may include the following:

- Unusual discharge at any time in the cycle
- Itching, stinging, swelling, or redness
- Sores of any kind, including blisters or warts
- Any unpleasant odor

If you do note any of these symptoms, you should be seen and diagnosed by a health-care practitioner.

PRIMARY FERTILITY SIGNS

Let's look at some of the physiological signs that your body sends out when it is most fertile.

Waking Body Temperature

While we rest at night, our body temperature drops from our active, daytime temperature of approximately 98.7°F. For the purposes of fertility, there are two distinct phases to our waking body temperature (also called basal body temperature or BBT). If a woman measures her waking temperature when her body is menstruating or getting ready to ovulate, it will normally register somewhere between 97°F and 97.7°F. Once the ovary has released the egg, however, women experience an increase in their waking body temperature, which rises to about 97.8°F or higher.

Progesterone, a hormone that is important for the regulation of ovulation and menstruation, is released at ovulation. As your progesterone level increases, your waking body temperature rises. When you measure your waking temperature at mid-cycle, that extra degree or so in temperature indicates that ovulation has already occurred. Your body is releasing the hormones needed to prepare your uterus to nurture a fertilized egg.

Checking Your Waking Body Temperature: The tool you will use to check your waking body temperature is a basal body temperature thermometer (sold at drugstores). This thermometer is not designed for measuring fever; it is calibrated specifically for calculating and charting your waking body temperature. The very first thing you should do upon waking, even before you sit up or move around, is take your temperature. Try to take your temperature at the same time each day and use the same part of your body, such as your mouth, each time. On your fertility chart, note the time of day of your temperature reading (see "How to Chart" on page 15).

Cervical Fluid

Your waking body temperature is only one fertility sign. It tells you whether you are ovulating at all, which is good to know. But since your temperature rises *after* ovulation, it is important to look at other fertility signs that can help you to time intercourse. If you wait until your ovary has released an egg, you may be too late. Cervical fluid (also called cervical mucus) provides one additional clue. The other is cervical position, which is discussed on page 12.

Throughout the course of your menstrual cycle, your cervix produces fluids in a regular, predictable pattern. (They are different from the lubrication that you notice during sexual arousal.) While every woman has her own unique cycle, there are certain times of the month when cervical fluid changes.

Once your menstrual flow ends, you won't notice any cervical fluid. Then after a few days of dryness and about a week before ovulation, your mucus pattern will change. You will notice the return of cervical fluid, which will usually be sticky or gummy. It can be white or a bit yellowish. After another few days, the fluid will become creamier, more like white or yellowish hand lotion.

Your Most Fertile Cervical Fluid: The slippery, stretchy fluid that marks your most fertile days usually arrives around day ten (remember that the exact day varies from one woman to the next). It is often a clear fluid, like egg white, but it can be streaked or even opaque. You may notice a round, wet spot in your underwear during this time, and your vagina will feel more lubricated.

On average, fertile cervical fluid lasts for three days and is a result of a boost in estrogen levels. Younger women often experience five days of this fertile fluid, while older women may have just one or two days. Once your estrogen drops and progesterone arrives (and your temperature starts to rise), the fertile fluid dries up within a day. Your most fertile day is the last day of the stretchy mucus. If you never experience stretchy or egg white–like mucus, your most fertile day is the last day of the wettest cervical mucus.

Sperm can live longer in fertile cervical mucus—up to five days—than in regular cervical fluid. The fertile mucus contains nutrients for the sperm to help it fertilize the egg. The pH level of fertile cervical fluid matches that of semen, an additional protectant for the sperm.

After your most fertile cervical fluid days, usually days ten to thirteen if you experience three days of stretchy fluid, your mucus changes again. It may disappear entirely, or become dry and sticky or quite thick. Any of these conditions makes it difficult for sperm to swim and reach the uterus. To maximize your chance of conception, have sex at the beginning of and throughout the time of your most stretchy cervical fluid.

Sex and Cervical Fluid: Sexual lubrication, the fluids secreted when you are sexually aroused, can mask cervical fluid. Be sure to check your cervical fluid when you are not sexually aroused. Semen looks a bit different from cervical fluid. It's more foamy or rubbery than any stage of cervical fluid and it dries more quickly. To learn the difference between semen and cervical fluid, place a small amount of semen between your thumb and index finger and rub them together. Semen usually does not have the stretchy quality of fertile cervical fluid.

Checking Your Cervical Fluid: Check your cervical fluid to gauge what is happening on each day of your fertility cycle. To do this, wipe yourself with a tissue from front to back and note how easily the tissue slides. Note your vaginal sensations as well. Do you feel dry? Wet? Sticky? Is there any discharge? What color is it?

Maintaining Your Cervical Fluid: Make sure to drink plenty of water or other hydrating beverages, which may actually boost the amount of cervical fluid you produce. Steer clear of decongestants and antihistamines, which can reduce the amount of mucus you produce.

Cervical Position

Like your cervical mucus and waking body temperature, your cervix will also change throughout your menstrual cycle. There is a subtle progression throughout the cycle. At the beginning, your cervix will feel firm and low. Gradually, as you move toward ovulation and your body prepares for a possible pregnancy, it will become softer, higher, and more open.

As you approach ovulation, your cervix will become wet with fertile fluid and rise to provide a wider "gate" for the sperm to pass through on their way to the uterus. Once ovulation has passed and you approach menstruation, the cervix reverses course, dropping lower as it becomes firmer, drier, and more closed.

Checking Your Cervix: By simply inserting your finger into your vagina and touching your cervix, you can discern these subtle changes. Not every woman is comfortable with putting a finger up her vagina and feeling around for changes. Take a deep breath and relax. Think of it this way: your finger is much, much smaller than the full-term baby that will use your vagina as its path into the wide world. Getting comfortable with the anatomy of fertility now can be a first step in making the mental transition from potential parent to expectant parent.

You will want to check your cervix during a few cycles to detect how it changes throughout the month, except while you are menstruating. Check at the same time each day, when you are unlikely to have a full bowel. Right after a shower is convenient for many women. Wash your hands thoroughly first. Checking while you're in a squat position is easiest, but you may choose to check while sitting on the toilet or with one foot up on the toilet lid.

Slide one finger into your vagina until it touches your cervix. Use the length of your finger as a guide to determine how high and how wet your cervix is. Press gently. Is it firm like the tip of your nose or finger? Or is it soft like your earlobe or lips? Finally, feel for the opening to begin to understand how your cervix feels when it is open and when it is closed.

Sex and Your Cervix: Intercourse can be uncomfortable during the postovulatory phase of your menstrual cycle, when your cervix is in the dropped or low position. Your partner's penis may actually come in contact with your cervix at this time. There is no reason for concern if this contact happens now or while you're pregnant. It is a natural part of sex.

When your cervix is low, you may experience discomfort in a straddle position, particularly if you are on top of your partner. This position, similar to squatting, pushes your cervix down even lower.

SECONDARY FERTILITY SIGNS

The signals for ovulation described earlier—fertile cervical mucus, cervical position, and waking body temperature—are considered the most reliable. But many women also experience secondary signals of ovulation, all perfectly normal, including the following:

- Breast sensitivity or tenderness
- Mid-cycle spotting or staining
- Increased energy level
- Pain in the ovaries—a dull pain as the follicle swells and a sharp one as the ovary releases the egg
- Abdominal bloating
- Increased libido
- Full or swollen vulva

OTHER METHODS OF PREDICTING OVULATION

There are kits and fertility monitors that can help you determine when you're about to ovulate.

Ovulation Predictor Kits: Available at any drugstore, an ovulation predictor kit (OPK) works like a home pregnancy test, but it measures the luteinizing hormone (LH) surge, which occurs right before ovulation. This hormonal surge triggers the release of a mature egg from one of the ovary's follicles. What kits do not tell you is whether or not you have actually ovulated. The idea is to pee on the little stick a day or so before you expect to ovulate. This tool helps you to time sex with your most fertile day or days.

Some women have an LH surge that lasts less than ten hours. If you are testing your LH just once a day, you could miss the surge. Other women have an LH level peak that is too low for the kit to detect. In addition to these limitations, the kit may show a hormonal surge when the cervical fluid is no longer optimal.

Fertility Monitors: The most popular fertility monitor is probably the Clearblue Easy Fertility Monitor, a palm-size electronic device that uses a urine test to monitor your fertility. A little computer analyzes your estrogen and LH levels and tells you when you are in the peak phase of your cycle. When used correctly, the monitor can accurately predict ovulation about one to two days before it occurs.

Salivary Ferning Test: This test predicts ovulation by looking at the amount of sodium in your saliva. As you approach ovulation, your saliva forms a distinct fernlike pattern, which you can see with the small microscope included in the kit. This is available at drugstores.

Ultrasound: If you seek fertility treatments such as intrauterine insemination or in vitro fertilization, most health-care providers will check for signs of ovulation by using ultrasound.

CHARTING YOUR FERTILITY CYCLE

While kits and monitors can help you identify your fertile days, you will get the most comprehensive information about your fertility cycle by charting your fertility signs. Keeping track of the physical changes that your body goes through each month helps you understand your fertility cycle and offers a methodical way for you to track any changes that may occur over longer periods of time, rather than during a single cycle.

The three primary fertility signs—waking body temperature, cervical fluid, and cervical position—are highly accurate and effective methods for identifying a woman's most and least fertile phases. Taken together with the secondary fertility signs, this system of understanding female fertility is known as the Fertility Awareness Method (FAM). It is empowering, involves little more than daily observation, and is completely natural. Here, in your own hands, is the knowledge you need to understand your reproductive health and your general gynecological health, too.

How to Chart

To get started, sit down with a sheet of blank paper and a pen. You will be making a landscape-shaped graph. Across the top, list cycle days 1 through 30. On the left side of the paper (the *y*-axis), begin about halfway up, and write a series of temperatures, beginning with 97 at the bottom and ending with 99 degrees at the top, each number increasing by a tenth of a degree (97.0, 97.1, 97.2, 97.3, etc.). There will be twenty-one numbers. Using a ruler, draw horizontal and vertical lines to make the grid, creating a space to mark your temperature for each day of your cycle. Below the temperature grid, leave some space to note the primary and secondary fertility signs discussed earlier. You may want to make a few copies of your blank chart before you begin charting.

Each day, record your waking temperature on the chart and make notes about the fertility signs you experience.

Here are a few questions to ask yourself as you begin to chart:

- Vaginal sensation—am I dry, sticky, or wet?
- Is there any cervical fluid present? If so, what does it look like today?
- Do I notice any ovulatory sensations or pain?
- How does my cervix feel?
- How is my energy level? Do I feel particularly tired or sick?
- Is today a period day? How heavy is the flow each day? What does the blood of my menstrual flow look like?
- Am I experiencing any signs of PMS or stress?
- Is travel or any other experience impacting my cycle?

The first day of your period is officially day one. On that day, you may experience heavy, red flow, as well as headache, cramps, and a foggy brain. As you move into post-flow days, you might write things like, "Sticky cervical fluid, light spotting." And as ovulation approaches and your cervical fluid changes, your notes might say, "Sticky white morning, creamy white afternoon, more cold and wet as the day went on. Sudden, sharp pain on left side on day 16."

Adding the Cover Line

As you now know, your basal body temperature rises after one of your ovaries has released an egg. Most women will see a significant change in their waking body temperature that corresponds to the release of the egg and subsequent burst of progesterone. Adding a cover line to your chart will help you visualize your temperature shift and ovulation. The following steps will guide you:

1. As you note your daily temperature, also note when your temperature rises at least 0.2°F above the previous day. For many women, this shift happens at about their cycle's two-week mark.
2. Count back six days from the day your temperature first shifted 0.2°F. Circle each of those six readings with a colored pen. Pick the highest of these temperatures, and make a mark on the chart 0.1°F above that.
3. Using a ruler, draw a line all the way across your chart at the level of the mark. This is your cover line.

UNDERSTANDING YOUR CHART

The cover line helps you to see two phases: preovulation, or the follicular phase, and postovulation, or the luteal phase. By focusing on the cover line, your eye can distinguish between the two phases and focus less on the daily ups and downs of your temperature. Over time, you will know how your chart usually looks during each fertility cycle and how to interpret any numbers that seem unusually high or low.

In the follicular phase, estrogen is the dominant hormone. In this phase, most women experience temperatures between 97°F and 97.5°F. The follicular phase lasts anywhere from twelve to fifteen days and varies from woman to woman.

In the luteal phase, progesterone is the dominant hormone. In this phase, your temperature increases by at least 0.4°F and stays elevated until your period starts, usually twelve to fifteen days after your ovulation date.

Identifying Your Peak Fertile Days

Your most fertile day is considered the last day that you experience one or more of these indicators: lubricative vaginal sensation (that wet, slippery feeling, whether or not there is any cervical fluid); mid-cycle spotting; or fertile cervical fluid (slippery and stretchy, like egg white).

Your peak day will most likely be the day before ovulation, but it can also occur on the day of ovulation. It will arrive a day or two before your waking or basal body temperature (BBT) shifts upward. Do not wait for your BBT to rise before you have sex. (Of course, you can always have sex again once your BBT does rise, just in case.)

If you are tracking your cervical fluid in order to achieve pregnancy, the day when your cervical fluid is the longest, most like egg white, and the stretchiest is your peak day. This most-stretchy-egg-white day is likely to occur a day or so before your thermal shift and is an excellent indicator of your peak fertility day or days.

Some women do not experience slippery or stretchy cervical fluid. Their cervical fluid may be creamy or smooth or feel like lotion. If you fall into this category, count the last day of your wettest fertile cervical fluid. (You will know your pattern of cervical fluid once you have been charting your fertility cycle for a few months.)

Once you have identified your peak fertility day, mark this day on your chart with brightly colored ink. Next, mark the four consecutive days that follow as day 1, 2, 3, 4. You are generally considered unlikely to conceive beginning on the evening of day four, as long as wetness does not reappear during this four-day count. After a few months of charting, you will know precisely when to time intercourse. Timing it to the days leading up to and during ovulation is the key.

The Impact of Stress on Your Peak Day

For most women, the wet vaginal sensations and any cervical fluid will dry up after the BBT rises, which is normally postovulation. What if you experience wet cervical fluid or wet vaginal sensations after your BBT rises? This may mean that you have not yet ovulated and progesterone has not yet been released. If this pattern occurs every month, it could also be a sign of stress, illness, or polycystic ovarian syndrome (see page 27).

Am I Pregnant?

If you do become pregnant, your temperature will do one of three things:

- Remain elevated for more than eighteen days once you enter the luteal phase.
- Remain high for three days longer than the longest luteal phase you have previously recorded.
- Be triphasic—that is, your temperature will increase as you move from the follicular to the luteal phase, then again from the luteal phase to pregnancy, and a third time during the luteal phase after implantation.

If your chart looks like stair steps, or you notice one of these signs, give your obstetrician/gynecologist a call.

GOING OFF THE PILL OR OTHER HORMONES, AND THE RETURN OF OVULATION

The birth control pill, known as "the Pill," is a combined oral contraceptive pill. This birth control method uses a combination of the estrogen estradiol and the progestogen progestin. This pill inhibits female fertility if it is taken orally every day. Over one hundred million women worldwide use the Pill to control fertility. Basically, a birth control pill tricks your hormonal or endocrine system into thinking you are pregnant every month. As a result, the Pill affects every aspect of your reproductive system, including ovulation, which the Pill prevents. By controlling the hormones that define your fertility system, the Pill also moderates or completely eliminates the secondary fertility signs. It can also cause unusual BBT readings, such as false high temperatures or temperatures that do not seem to be in sync with the quality of cervical fluid. And the Pill may cause any of the following disruptions:

- Heavier or thicker bleeding
- Lighter or thinner bleeding
- Spotting in the luteal phase
- Shorter luteal phases
- Changes in your cervical fluid, including an absence of cervical fluid, an unchanged cervical fluid throughout the cervical fluid phase, or cervical fluid that is not of fertile quality.

When you stop taking the Pill or another form of hormonal birth control, thus stopping the hormone suppression that makes them so effective, there is no accurate method to predict when your cycle will return to its natural rhythm and pattern. Some women may ovulate almost immediately, within a couple of weeks, while others may experience a delay of months or even years. This variation is a function of the type and dosage of the Pill used, as well as a woman's unique physiology.

Charting and the Pill

Talk with your health-care provider about the best time to come off the Pill. Ideally, you want to begin charting on the first day of menstruation after you've stopped taking it. Record day one as the first day of bleeding. If that is not possible, you may begin to chart mid-cycle. Begin recording your temperature and checking your cervical fluid as soon as possible. If you begin charting mid-cycle, record the date and temperature of the first day of your next period as day one on a new chart. Charting when coming off of any hormonal interference with your fertility system can be confusing. Note any of the disruptions to your fertility signs on your chart. Give your body time to adjust and return to its natural fertility rhythm again. Be aware too that your body has aged as time has passed and your new rhythm may return exactly as it once was or it may take on a new character.

The Myth of Day Fourteen

Couples may inadvertently prevent pregnancy by subscribing to the myth of day fourteen. That is, many woman attempting to achieve pregnancy believe they ovulate on day fourteen of every menstrual cycle. You may, in fact, ovulate on day fourteen, but it is not a given and here's why: While many women experience a twenty-eight-day menstrual cycle, plenty of others do not. Their cycle may be as short as twenty-four days or as long as thirty-six. Over time, a woman's cycle can change and become longer or shorter. Fertility signs also change and may vary slightly from month to month.

A menstrual cycle of between twenty-four and thirty-six days is considered normal. The reality of your own cycle may be much different. Ovulation may occur much earlier than day fourteen or much later. As noted earlier, the key is to have intercourse on the days leading up to and during ovulation. Though an egg is only viable for twelve to twenty-four hours, sperm can live inside a woman's reproductive tract for up to five days. A woman can get pregnant from an act of intercourse occurring anytime from about five days prior to ovulation to even two days after. This means a woman can get pregnant during any given cycle for about seven cycle days. By charting primary and secondary fertility signs, each woman will discover her own unique rhythm for her cycle, her own day of ovulation, and her number of most fertile days.

The Pill contributes to the myth of day fourteen because it manipulates the body's hormones to maintain a fertility cycle of twenty-eight days. Whether a woman naturally has a twenty-eight-day cycle or not cannot be determined until she removes hormonal contraceptive interventions from her life and begins charting to determine her own cycle. (The myth of day fourteen is also responsible for many unplanned pregnancies, because some women assume that they cannot get pregnant on any other day.)

Now that you are well informed, you can help debunk the myth of day fourteen for others who may benefit from knowing this critical detail about fertility.

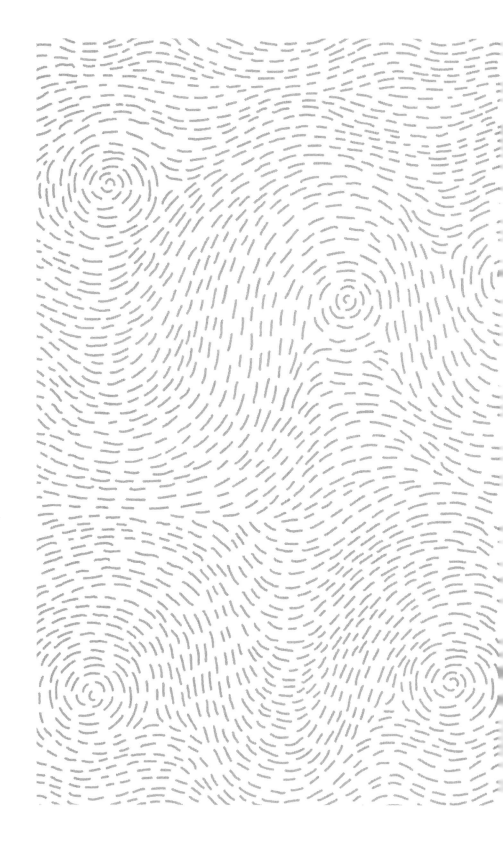

CHAPTER TWO

Maximize Your Chances of Getting Pregnant

Are you leading a fertility-friendly lifestyle? Before you begin trying to conceive, it is important to step back and take an honest look at your life. You may love the way you live now, but you probably need to make a few changes in order to support your fertility. That is not to say that all fun should be removed from your life the moment you start trying to conceive. But it is time to think about the lifestyle choices that are most important to you and your partner.

CULTIVATING A HEALTHY LIFESTYLE

Your body is the health and wellness system for a future embryo, providing it with all the nourishment it needs for development. This is true from day one of any pregnancy and even a few months before conception. Keep in mind that once a sperm penetrates an egg, an embryo's heart and nervous system begin developing almost immediately. The lifestyle choices you make while trying to get pregnant may be as important as what you do while you are pregnant.

Tobacco, recreational drugs, and alcohol are linked to fertility problems, miscarriages, and birth defects. To improve your fertility, it's advisable to give them all up.

The following questions suggest other changes you may need to make:

- Are you a healthy weight for your body type? Roughly 12 percent of fertility issues stem from weight problems—because a woman is over- or underweight.
- Do you exercise regularly? Regular exercise helps control blood sugar levels, fights inflammation, and relieves stress.
- Are you getting enough sleep? You already know that getting enough sleep is important for brain function. Lack of sleep can alter your hormonal balance, lead to irregular menstrual cycles, and affect ovulation.

- How much caffeine do you consume each day? While studies on caffeine and fertility are inconclusive, we know that caffeine can increase stress and anxiety levels and decrease the flow of blood to the uterus, which may negatively impact implantation. It is best to limit your caffeine intake when trying to conceive to just one or two cups of coffee in the morning. Tea, which offers beneficial antioxidants and has less caffeine per serving than coffee, can be a good alternative. Be mindful of caffeine in other sources, such as energy drinks, chocolate, over-the-counter medicine, and gum.

Medications, Vitamins, and Herbal Medicines

Keep an eye on the medications, vitamins, and herbal medicines that you take regularly. As discussed earlier, some medications, such as antihistamines and cough medicine, can reduce or dry up cervical mucus. Pain relievers can reduce blood flow to the uterus. Anti-inflammatories, such as Advil and Aleve, can stop ovulation entirely and have also been shown to reduce cervical mucus.

If you are taking birth control pills, many doctors recommend waiting at least one full menstrual cycle after you've gone off the Pill before trying to conceive.

Before your next visit to your obstetrician/gynecologist (ob-gyn), prepare a list of all over-the-counter and prescription medications you are taking, as well as any vitamins, supplements, or herbal medicines. Studies on many vitamin supplements and herbal medicines are limited, and their effects on fertility may not be known. Have a frank discussion with your health-care provider about your fertility goals to determine the best choices for you.

Women should begin taking a prenatal vitamin and men should begin taking a multivitamin three months before trying to conceive.

Concerns for Men

Like women, men can also benefit from improving their lifestyle. The quantity and quality of sperm are the main reproductive issues that men face.

The Importance of Vitamins

A vitamin deficiency may be implicated in a low sperm count, which is a common concern for men. There are millions of sperm sent into the vagina during intercourse, but the odds of one finding an egg are quite low. A low sperm count is defined as fewer than twenty million sperm per milliliter of semen.

In some cases of low sperm count, mild cases of zinc deficiency have been implicated. Studies also suggest that a deficiency in vitamin A or B, or selenium may be the problem. (Almost half of a man's selenium supply is located in the testicles and seminal ducts.)

Arginine, a nonessential amino acid, can help increase sperm count and motility in some men. For men with marginal sperm counts, limiting the frequency of ejaculation can also help. A maximum frequency of once every forty-eight hours is recommended.

The Impact of Stress

Most of us live with some degree of stress. Pressures from our professional lives, difficult in-laws, traffic jams, holidays, and the obligations and expectations associated with them are all common causes of stress. Of course, dealing with infertility also carries with it its own stress. Our physiological response to stress—sweaty palms, restless sleep, rapid heartbeat—are familiar enough. But there is another aspect to stress that is worth examining when considering fertility.

When your body engages in the stress response, it overproduces adrenaline and cortisol. In prehistoric times, these hormones were critical; they gave us the speed we needed to escape predators or fight an enemy with unusual strength. Adrenaline and cortisol protected us from harm and allowed us to live another day.

When looking at these hormones in the context of fertility, the fight-or-flight response that was so important to our forebears takes on a different meaning. Activation of the adrenal glands, and the subsequent overproduction of adrenaline and cortisol, interferes with the production of hormones that are important for fertility, namely follicle-stimulating hormone (FSH) and luteinizing hormone (LH). The decrease in FSH and LH in turn decreases the hormones progesterone, testosterone, and estrogen, all of which manage the process of an egg's fertilization and implantation. Chronic physiological and psychological stress can also stop ovulation and menstruation.

Men are not immune from the negative effects of stress. Lower sperm counts, decreased sperm motility and quality, and a higher percentage of abnormal sperm are all scientifically confirmed effects of stress in men. Studies have shown that full fertility is restored when the stress disappears. Reduce stress and you may be able to reduce or even reverse a fertility problem.

HOW TO COPE WITH STRESS NATURALLY

Take a hard look at how you manage stress in your everyday life. Some women respond to stress by doing a little retail therapy. Others react by eating significantly more or less. Some drink alcohol to take the edge off.

Are there healthful changes you can make to improve your response to stress? Meditation, moderate exercise, singing to your favorite music, cooking a favorite meal, and talk therapy are gentle ways to work through stress. All of these methods can be used at any stage of your menstrual cycle to promote relaxation. Over time, you will develop a new awareness of your stress triggers and how to cope with stress in a fertility-positive way. This focus on your well-being has a bonus: you will begin to develop a new connection with your physical self.

As noted in the discussion about charting (see page 14), the menstrual cycle has three distinct fertile phases: menstruation, preovulation, and post-ovulation. There are unique hormonal changes that occur at each phase. Since stress also triggers a hormonal response, how you respond to stress during each phase of your cycle can be fine-tuned to optimize fertility.

Menstruation

When trying to get pregnant, women tend to view menstruation as a sign that they did not achieve pregnancy in a given cycle. Give yourself permission to feel sad if you do start your period. Use this time to rest, relax, and rejuvenate your sense of well-being. Find a quiet spot in your home and light a candle. Think of one thing that you are thankful for—your partner, your career, your dog, a delicious meal. This can help reset your mind to the peaceful energy of a new beginning. Day one is the start of a new cycle, so chill out: sleep a little more and enjoy the quiet for a few days while your attention is turned inward.

A Breathing Exercise to Reduce Stress During Menstruation

Sit comfortably, either in a chair with your feet touching the ground, or on the floor. Close your eyes. Inhale deeply, allowing your ribs and your belly to expand. Count to five as you continue to breathe in. See if you can feel your breath move through your body. Then as you exhale, pull your abdomen in and push any negative thoughts out and away from your body. After a few minutes of breathing this way, shift the focus of your breath to your core—the area below your diaphragm, cradled by your hips. With your breath, begin to warm up your core, the center of your feminine energy. Visualize the breath nourishing your uterus, providing it with the energy, light, and strength it needs to begin life.

Preovulation

Estrogen dominates now and increases your sense of well-being. You may feel sexier now and more inclined to engage in activities outside of your home. Before ovulation is a great time to connect with your partner and friends and get a little exercise. If you enjoy a glass of wine with dinner, now is a safe time to indulge, as your risk of pregnancy is very low.

A Breathing Exercise to Reduce Stress During Preovulation

Use the same breathing exercise for this phase that you used during menstruation.

Once your core is warm and your negative thoughts have been pushed out, try to entertain thoughts of gathering or embracing. Collect the energy your body will need to become pregnant. Imagine your family and friends—those who will support you during your pregnancy—around you. In your mind, hold your partner's hand. Visualize your breath nourishing your uterus, providing it with the energy, light, and strength it needs to begin life.

Ovulation and Possible Implantation

The pressure to have sex at just the right time on just the right day can be nerve-wracking for each partner and place a great deal of strain on your relationship. Stress on your male partner can negatively impact his performance. Because estrogen, FSH, and LH increase at ovulation, you may experience a sense of overall well-being. Rather than pressure your partner for sex at this time—which creates stress—think back to the times in your relationship when sex came easily and naturally and did not feel forced by circumstances. What did you do in the days and hours leading up to having sex? What did your partner do? Try and re-create that relaxed, spontaneous atmosphere now. Sex should be fun and spirited, now more than ever, and a way to physically connect with your partner.

A Visualization Exercise for Ovulation and Postovulation

Use the same breathing exercise for this phase that you used during menstruation and preovulation. Once your core is warm and you have mentally gathered your family, friends, and partner around you, visualize the fertilized egg arriving in your uterus and finding a place there to grow and develop. Allow yourself to remember the steps you have taken and are continuing to take to nourish and support an embryo. Say yes to the changes you have made and are continuing to make to bring a new life into this world. Visualize your breath nourishing your uterus, providing it with the energy, light, and strength it needs to begin life.

TESTS AND NATURAL TREATMENTS TO CONSIDER

It's a good idea to have your annual physical exam before you start down the fertility path. This will provide your physician and ob-gyn with basic information about your overall health before they recommend any testing related to fertility.

With this basic information and your charting, your physician or ob-gyn can tell you if you or your partner may have a physiological problem that is reducing your fertility.

There are a number of preliminary tests for you and your partner to discuss with your health-care provider. These include cultures for infections, including sexually transmitted diseases. Postcoital tests check to see that sperm are getting where they need to go. A semen analysis evaluates the number, movement, and shape of the sperm. A hysterosalpingogram and a hysteroscopy use different technologies to examine the lining of the uterus and fallopian tubes to make sure there are no blockages, fibroids, or anything else that might be interfering with the egg's journey to and implantation in the uterus. Hormone tests are conducted on specific days of a woman's menstrual cycle to look at the levels of estradiol, progesterone, FSH, LH, and testosterone. Men need to have their hormones tested as well, including testosterone, FSH, and LH. The following medical conditions are some that your ob-gyn may want to rule out through testing.

Hypothyroidism

Low levels of certain hormones produced by your thyroid are symptoms of hypothyroidism, a condition that can interfere with the release of an egg from your ovary. In addition, some of the underlying causes of hypothyroidism, including certain autoimmune or pituitary disorders, may impair fertility. A complete thyroid panel can confirm whether or not your thyroid is operating normally.

Anovulation and Polycystic Ovarian Syndrome

Many health-care providers now believe that polycystic ovarian syndrome (PCOS) is one of the most common causes of infertility. When a woman has PCOS, the ovaries are unable to create a fully mature egg and none are released. The follicles in the ovaries turn into fluid-filled sacs known as cysts. Without the release of an egg, progesterone is not released and menstruation becomes irregular or stops. The cysts then make androgens, the so-called male hormones, which compounds the situation.

Symptoms of PCOS can vary from woman to woman. They include an excessive quantity of the hormones LH and FSH, high blood insulin levels, male-pattern facial and body hair, and acne. About half of all women diagnosed with PCOS are overweight. The extra weight can stem from insulin resistance—a defect in the way the body processes sugar—which can disrupt a woman's hormone balance. But some women have no symptoms at all.

If you think you may have PCOS, ask your health-care provider to check the levels of your testosterone, FSH, LH, and DHEA (the hormone dehydroepiandrosterone), and be sure to ask for a complete blood glucose panel, including insulin levels.

There are three steps to returning to good health after a diagnosis of PCOS:

1. **Lose weight.** In numerous studies, a loss of 5 percent of a woman's weight can have a significant impact on PCOS. This modest weight loss can immediately improve the body's sensitivity to insulin, improve menstrual regularity and ovulation, and reduce acne.
2. **Eat fewer carbohydrates.** A diet that is lower in carbohydrates can have a direct and immediate impact for women with PCOS by keeping blood sugar and insulin under control and reducing food cravings. Women with PCOS should eat more healthy proteins and fats. (See Chapter 3.)

3. **Take the right medication.** Two classes of drugs traditionally used to treat diabetes can also improve blood sugar and promote ovulation in women with PCOS: metformin and thiazolidinediones. The first cuts down the liver's need to release stored glucose; the second lowers insulin and androgen levels and improves ovulation.

Endometriosis

When a woman has endometriosis, the tissue that usually lines the inside of the uterus instead grows outside of it. This misplaced tissue can develop anywhere in the abdominal cavity or within cysts in the ovaries. The condition is unpredictable and may remain in a small area or spread through the abdomen. Symptoms include heavy or disabling menstrual cramps, chronic pelvic or lower back pain, painful urination, spotting between periods, pain with intercourse, and infertility. Hormonal therapy or surgery is used to treat this condition.

Luteinized Unruptured Follicle Syndrome

Even if you have all of the classic signs of ovulation, your ovaries may not release an egg. One potential cause is a condition called luteinized unruptured follicle syndrome (LUFS). It is estimated that up to 30 percent of all cases of unexplained infertility are due to LUFS. If your health-care provider suspects LUFS, an ultrasound can confirm the problem.

Premature Ovarian Failure

The condition in which a woman's ovaries stop producing eggs a decade or more before normal menopause is known as premature ovarian failure (POF). It may emerge suddenly or over a period of years. Symptoms are similar to those of menopause and include hot flashes, vaginal dryness, and lack of menstruation. A blood test repeated over a period of months on day three of your cycle to check FSH and estrogen will confirm POF. Women who have this condition often use donor eggs and in vitro fertilization to give birth.

TRADITIONAL CHINESE MEDICINE

Alternative therapies, particularly those of traditional Chinese medicine (TCM), have become increasingly popular. As a means to achieving pregnancy, they present less invasive alternatives to Western medicine.

TCM focuses on specific problems and aims to provide relief for the symptoms associated with these conditions. It also seeks to maintain and support optimal health and wellness, and to prevent problems from developing in the first place.

TCM is based on the ancient Chinese belief that humans are microcosms of the universe; we are connected with nature, and shaped by its forces. According to TCM, the organs, tissues, and other parts of the human body have distinct functions, but they are also all interconnected. When a person is healthy, her bodily functions are all in harmony. When she is sick, they are out of balance. TCM practitioners try to find the causes of any imbalances.

Underlying TCM are the concepts of yin and yang, two opposite but complementary forces that shape the natural world and all forms of life. The characteristics of yin and yang are often likened to fire and water. Like water, yin is cold and heavy, passive, and yielding. It is often described as feminine energy. Yang is like fire, bright and aggressive, hot and quick. Yang is often described as masculine energy. Within yin, there is a kernel of yang; within yang, there is a kernel of yin. Each needs the other, and each is present in the other. It is the balance between the energies, or qi, that matters.

Qi is the energy or life force that enlivens every cell in our bodies. TCM looks at our bodies as a series of interconnected energies that flow in patterns. This energy flows throughout every part of the body, invigorating and empowering our organs and the processes that link them. According to TCM, qi flows through the body along meridians or energy channels. These channels have been mapped by TCM practitioners for more than two thousand years. The insertion of needles at different points along these meridians (acupuncture) or the application of force along these meridians (acupressure) produces measurable effects on your body's organs and systems.

The qi that flows through our bodies is the same qi present in every other part of the universe. Air, water, plants, and animals all share the same qi. A yin-yang imbalance leads to disharmony in your qi energy. To correct any imbalances, practitioners of TCM use a combination of food therapy, massage, therapeutic exercises, medicinal herbs, and acupuncture.

Western medicine also recognizes the importance of balance in the human body. Homeostasis is a state of equilibrium between different elements of an organism or group. In humans, it's the body's ability to maintain its biochemistry by continually adjusting to the demands placed upon it, both internally and externally.

Let's use the example of headaches to clarify how Western and Eastern medicine differ in approach. Using Western medicine, you might treat the symptoms of the headache by using a pain reliever, such as Advil. This approach provides relief but does not get at the root cause of the problem. So if the headache persists, you would see your doctor, who in turn might order tests to determine whether your headache is a symptom of a bigger problem. Further treatment might be prescribed.

For the same headache, practitioners of TCM would attempt to discover any imbalance that is creating the symptom. Instead of a pill to relieve symptoms or tests to check for signs of a bigger problem, the practitioner would read your pulse and check your tongue to understand the state of your organs and meridians. With this information, the practitioner would diagnose a deficiency in one or more of your energetic systems. He or she might prescribe herbs, dietary changes, or acupuncture to bring your organs and energy systems back into balance.

This fundamental difference between Western and Eastern approaches—treating the energetic health underlying an organ versus treating an organ itself—is important to keep in mind when seeking support for infertility. Western medicine looks for problems in the ovaries and other reproductive organs, tests hormone levels, and treats any problems or symptoms. Eastern medicine looks for imbalances in the network of organs, hormones, and energy systems that prevent a woman's body from conceiving. TCM investigates every aspect of your health history and habits, and seeks to restore balance.

With regard to fertility, Western and Eastern medicine can be complementary. For example, TCM alone cannot help you conceive if you have a structural problem such as fibroids or a blocked fallopian tube. But TCM can support your return to optimum health by restoring your qi energy and yin-yang balance after you have resolved these issues with Western medicine. In fact, alternative medicine practices such as acupuncture are used by more and more women who have experienced difficulty when trying to conceive. Many IVF clinics now offer acupuncture as a service for their patients. Acupuncture can increase blood flow to the uterus and ovaries, stimulate hormone production, tamp down stress hormones, and increase sperm count and motility.

There have been no studies on whether Chinese herbal medicine improves infertility. However, Chinese herbs are used to increase cervical mucus, increase blood circulation, help reach and maintain a healthy waking body temperature, lengthen a short postovulation phase, and improve the quality and quantity of sperm. Women with PCOS or other hormonal issues may want to try acupuncture treatments to stabilize the hormonal system.

If you do choose to follow traditional Chinese medicine as part of your fertility-positive efforts, there are other benefits as well. Acupuncture can be very effective at relieving stress and anxiety by freeing stagnant qi energy. Working along the meridians, on acupuncture points on the hands and feet, head, and ears—a treatment called "four gates"—is very effective for providing relaxation. (Many patients fall asleep during the treatment.) All women and men can benefit from the calming and relaxing effects of acupuncture on the nervous and neuroendocrine systems.

GENDER SELECTION WITH THE SHETTLES METHOD

For centuries, theories have been bandied about on how to select the gender of a hoped-for child. Positions, lotions, certain metals, and even the hair of a newt have been linked to gender selection according folk beliefs, old and modern.

Then in the 1970s, along came Dr. Landrum Shettles, who developed a sci-entifically based method to increase a couple's chances of choosing a child's gender. His book *How to Choose the Sex of Your Baby* (revised in 2006) is the source for couples seeking additional information on this topic.

The Fertility Awareness Method outlined in this chapter serves as a base-line for incorporating Shettle's principles of gender selection. The method is not foolproof, though. Shettles claims an 80 to 90 percent effectiveness rate for choosing boys and 75 to 80 percent for selecting girls when his methods are followed properly.

The fundamental principle on which the Shettles Method is based is that sperm determine what gender a baby will be. Male sperm carry the Y chro-mosome and female sperm carry the X chromosome. Male sperm are lighter, smaller, faster, and more fragile than their female counterparts. Female sperm tend to live longer than the male sperm.

What does this mean for the "fertility positive"? To weight your chances of having a boy, you should time sex to be as close to ovulation as possible. The lighter, faster male sperm in this scenario will reach the egg before the slower, heavier female sperm. On the other hand, if you want to try for a girl, time intercourse before ovulation but still during your fertile days.

Everything from environmental stress to a man's age may have an impact on the effectiveness of the Shettles Method. A number of different studies link environmental stress with an increase in female offspring. For example, men with low sperm counts tend to have more female sperm. Shettles theorizes that the same factors that cause low sperm count, such as drugs and toxins, also kill off more of the more fragile male sperm. Girls are born in higher numbers to couples who utilize IVF for pregnancy achievement. Female sperm are better at surviving the laboratory stresses that are involved in IVF.

On the other end of the spectrum, there is a tendency for younger couples to conceive more male babies than older couples. The higher sperm counts of younger men and the higher quality, more alkaline cervical fluid of younger women are thought to be the reasons. Similarly, couples who receive artificial insemination or intrauterine insemination are more likely to conceive males because these methods are timed as close to ovulation as possible.

MYTHS, URBAN LEGENDS, AND REAL SCIENCE

You've heard them all. Here's a quick primer to assure you that sometimes, a myth is just a myth.

Tight underwear reduces a man's sperm count.

False. As long as your partner wears pants over his underwear, the temperature of his scrotum will not be adversely affected, and his choice of underwear will have no impact on his sperm count.

Hot tubs reduce his sperm count.

True. Spending time in hot tubs and saunas heated over 100°F can heat sperm to levels that are too warm for their survival and as a result, decrease sperm counts. Your partner can play it safe by avoiding hot tubs for about three months before trying to conceive.

Bicycling reduces his sperm count, too.

Maybe. The combination of tight shorts, added heat from sweating in the scrotal area, and the constant bumping of the testes may contribute to reduced sperm numbers. If a man's sperm analysis is fine, proceed with this heart-healthy, stress-reducing activity. If not, it may be one more lifestyle change to consider while practicing positive fertility.

You should not use lubricants during sex if you are trying to get pregnant.

True. Almost all lubricants, from vegetable oil to petroleum jelly to saliva, can kill sperm. Recently, a new lubricant called Pre-Seed entered the market. It is designed to mimic the body's natural secretions and provide an optimal, pH-balanced environment for sperm.

Douches, vaginal sprays, and scented tampons are fertility friendly.

False. Douches alter the natural pH level of the vagina and ironically can lead to vaginal infections. Even worse, they can wash away cervical fluid, which sperm need for traveling through the cervix to the egg. Vaginal sprays and scented tampons contain chemicals that can cause a pH imbalance in the vagina or an allergic reaction. Do not use any of these while trying to conceive.

It does not matter what position you use during intercourse.

False. Yes, sex is sex and sex is the most direct path to pregnancy. But if your partner has a marginal sperm count, the missionary position is the best one for fertility. It allows for the deepest penetration of the penis, placing the sperm as close as possible to the cervix. Some clinicians also recommend remaining on your back after intercourse with your pelvis tilted up to allow the sperm some additional time to travel up the cervix.

It does not matter how much you weigh.

False. Maintaining a healthy weight and being in good general health is the first step to optimizing fertility. In order to ovulate, women should aim for about 20 percent body fat. Being overweight, with a much higher percentage of body fat, can cause an overproduction of estrogen and lead to delayed ovulation and irregular cycles. Being underweight can prevent ovulation altogether.

You can still drink your super-caffeinated beverage every morning.

False. Caffeine decreases blood flow to the uterus, which negatively impacts the body's ability to conceive and to nurture an embryo. For almost everyone, up to 90 milligrams of caffeine per day is considered safe. However, if you have been diagnosed with unexplained infertility or simply wish to naturally increase your fertility, eliminating or significantly reducing caffeine in your diet is a good idea.

It is safe to drink alcohol before you get pregnant.

False. No amount of alcohol is considered safe at any time during pregnancy and is one of the most common factors affecting fertility in men. While trying to conceive, it is best for you and your partner to reserve alcoholic drinks for special occasions and only during the menstruation and preovulation phases of each fertility cycle.

NOURISHING YOUR BODY BEFORE YOU START TRYING

From the moment of conception, your nutritional needs will change. Your body will become the cafeteria of life for the tiny cluster of cells that has begun to grow.

Most of us will not know the moment when we conceive. We learn this snippet of data somewhere down the line, after checking our BBT for a full cycle, or peeing on a stick or getting a blood test to confirm that we have, in fact, become pregnant. Because of this data lag, most health-care providers recommend that women who are trying to conceive begin a nutritional regimen that boosts fertility and provides the nutrients needed to support the very earliest development of a fetus.

Prenatal Vitamins and Multivitamins

Both partners involved in trying to conceive benefit from the addition of a multivitamin. Studies have shown that men who begin a vitamin regimen boost their immune system, their sperm count, and the quality and motility of their sperm. Women should start taking prenatal vitamins about three months before trying to conceive. They are specifically designed for women who hope to become or are pregnant, and provide the recommended levels of the nutrients most important for the early stage of life. In most cases, a prenatal vitamin will be the only vitamin needed.

Health-care practitioners recommend taking your vitamin with a meal, as vitamins taken with food have a higher absorption rate than those taken without.

Important Nutrients

Here, more specifically, are the nutrients your body needs.

The B Vitamins

The human body needs vitamin B9, often referred to as folic acid or folate, to synthesize and repair DNA. It aids rapid cell division and growth, which is especially important during pregnancy and early childhood. Good sources of B9 include liver; leafy green vegetables; legumes such as beans, lentils, and peas; and avocados and peanuts. Other B vitamins that are important for supporting fertility are B1 (thiamine), B5 (pantothenic acid), B6, and B12. A deficiency in vitamin B1 has been linked to anovulation. B2 supports estrogen metabolism and B5 supports the body's ability to synthesize and metabolize proteins, fats, and carbohydrates. Vitamin B6 helps the body produce progesterone and metabolize excess estrogen. B12 plays a key role in the normal functioning of the brain and nervous system and in the formation of blood. Good sources of B vitamins also include asparagus, dairy products, eggs, meat, nuts, salmon, shellfish, and sweet potatoes.

Vitamin A

An antioxidant, vitamin A is important during the production of male and female sex hormones, especially progesterone. Good sources of vitamin A include apricots, dairy products, dark green vegetables, eggs, fish, meat, and orange vegetables such as carrots, winter squashes, and yams.

Vitamin D

Another antioxidant, vitamin D supports the production of estrogen and the body's ability to absorb calcium. Good food sources include fish, shellfish, and fortified milk. Sunshine is an excellent source of vitamin D.

Calcium

Calcium helps build and maintain strong bones. It is also important for hormonal balance and proper blood clotting, and it supports sperm motility. Good sources of calcium include almonds, dairy products, flaxseed and oil, oily fish (such as bluefish, mackerel, and sardines), and shellfish.

Iron

Iron plays a key role in DNA replication and supports the egg's maturation prior to ovulation. Women normally require more iron than men because they naturally lose blood each month during menstruation. Good sources of iron include beans, blackstrap molasses, eggs, fortified cereal, poultry, pumpkin seeds and oil, red meat (such as beef and lamb), and tofu.

Manganese, Selenium, and Zinc

Manganese helps break down estrogen. Selenium is important for egg production, and zinc is vital for proper cell division and growth. All are also important factors for male fertility. Good sources include eggs, nuts, and whole grains.

Coenzyme Q10

Coenzyme Q10 (CoQ10) is essential for cell formation and improves blood flow. It is found in seminal fluid, where it improves motility. CoQ10 is difficult to get from food. A supplement is recommended.

Omega-3 and Omega-6 Fatty Acids

Fats are a form of stored energy and are critically important to support fertility and pregnancy. They are building blocks for hormones, and they can have powerful effects on the body, such as triggering inflammation or turning genes on and off. Recent research has demonstrated the importance of essential fatty acids (EFAs) in the formation of body tissue and brain development in the fetus. Our bodies cannot produce these fatty acids, so we must eat foods that contain them.

Most Americans eat enough omega-6s in the form of vegetable oils, such as corn, sunflower, safflower, and soybean oil. These oils are often used in packaged foods. Americans, however, don't eat enough foods rich in omega-3 fatty acids. Good sources of omega-3s include flax and chia seeds and their oils, as well as sea vegetables, eggs, and fatty fish such as salmon, sardines, and herring. Good sources of omega-6s include corn, dairy products, eggs, meat, and vegetable oils (such as, soybean, sunflower, and safflower).

Because fish is such a good source of omega-3 fatty acids, it is an important part of the fertility diet. But be aware that mercury, an industrial pollutant and heavy metal harmful to fertility and overall health, has entered our food supply through the foods we get from the ocean. It is still safe to eat most fish, but while attempting to conceive, it is recommended that you limit the types and amount of fish you eat. In general, the smaller the species of fish, the less likely it is to contain mercury.

For women who are attempting to conceive—as well as pregnant women, small children, and anyone with a compromised immune system–the Environmental Protection Agency recommends following these steps when choosing fish and shellfish. In order to be confident that you are reducing your exposure to the harmful effects of mercury:

1. Do not eat shark, swordfish, king mackerel, or tilefish. These top predators contain high, unsafe levels of mercury.
2. Eat two or three 6-ounce servings of fish per week. Five of the most commonly eaten fish that are low in mercury are shrimp, salmon, pollock (often used in prepackaged seafood products), and catfish. Canned light tuna is also low in mercury, but albacore tuna contains more mercury. So when choosing your two meals of fish and shellfish, you may eat up to 6 ounces (one average meal) of albacore tuna per week.
3. Check local advisories about the safety of fish caught by family and friends in your local lakes, rivers, and coastal areas. If no advice is available, eat up to 6 ounces per week of fish you catch from local waters, but don't consume any other fish during that week.

Good nutrition can correct all sorts of health imbalances, including those related to fertility. Eating well for fertility is generally similar to eating well for overall good health. Information on the dietary requirements for fertility is included in the next chapter.

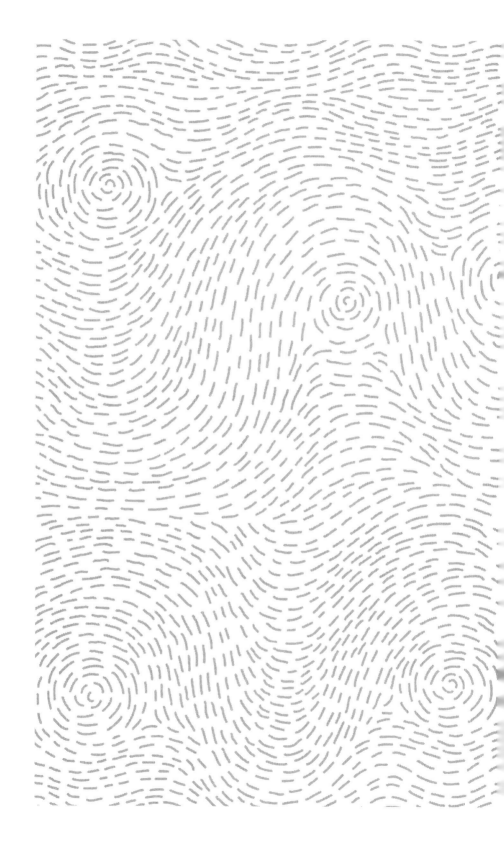

CHAPTER THREE

Getting Started on the Fertility Diet

Ever since we were kids, we have been told, "You are what you eat." Now that we are adults, common sense tells us that sentiment was right. Health is to a great extent the direct result of what we put into the machine that is our body. Medical research on any bodily function or system, including your reproductive system, supports the fact that how and what you eat is directly correlated with your health.

We eat at least three meals a day and usually a few snacks and beverages. The choices we make about what we put into our bodies each and every day can mean the difference between healthy and unhealthy, fertile and infertile. If you already eat a healthy diet, you may be familiar with many of the dietary choices that are beneficial for fertility. But keep in mind that eating and drinking for overall good health and eating and drinking for fertility, though similar in many ways, are not exactly the same. You need to eat for optimum health *and* to promote fertility.

THE SCIENCE BEHIND THE FERTILITY DIET

The eating strategy at the core of the fertility diet is the consumption of foods that are digested slowly, contain the highest levels of the nutrients, support general health, and boost fertility. The diet includes a balance of proteins, carbohydrates, and fats from a wide range of foods that promote wellness and fertility, while minimizing foods that are less beneficial.

Consuming foods from all food groups is important, but it is also important to choose those foods in each food group that are digested slowly. Foods that pass through your digestive system slowly keep blood sugar in the safe zone after you have eaten, and keep it there between meals. This work is done by two key hormones: insulin and glucagon. The trajectory of your blood sugar over the course of the day can make a difference to your health and your fertility.

The fertility diet seeks to diminish the peaks and valleys of blood sugar and insulin for two reasons: If you experience too many peaks or sugar highs, you can develop insulin resistance and increase your risk for type 2 diabetes, as well as other health problems. Reducing the peaks and valleys also reduces your risk of hormonal and ovulatory problems that impair fertility.

Insulin and glucagon work together to turn what you eat into a simple sugar known as glucose, which your cells use to perform their jobs properly. The main problem with foods that are digested quickly is that insulin and glucagon make this conversion rapidly. When too much sugar enters the bloodstream at once, the pancreas churns out more insulin to help tissues such as muscles absorb the glucose. When the pancreas senses the resulting decline in blood sugar, it slows the production of insulin and pushes up the production of glucagon. The liver then responds by releasing more glucose into the bloodstream to break down the glucagon. For overall good health, a fertility-positive diet that minimizes this rise and fall of blood sugar is the first task.

FOODS TO EAT AND FOODS TO AVOID

Foods that are digested slowly come from all food groups. What matters is how much the food has been altered from its original form. As an example, let's take an apple: If you eat a whole apple, you are eating all the nutrients of the apple's skin and the flesh. If you consume part of the apple, as juice or as fruit strips, you are benefiting nutritionally from only the juice, not the skin. Perhaps most important, the transformation of a whole apple into juice makes it more readily absorbed into the bloodstream.

The unprocessed apple has all of its nutrients intact and is digested slowly. The juice, when consumed by itself, provides less nutrition and is digested more rapidly, which can cause a spike in blood sugar. The same principle applies to just about any food, including carbohydrates.

Carbohydrates

Carbohydrates have gotten a bad rap because so many of the comfort foods in our diet are carbohydrates that are quickly transformed during digestion into glucose, which spikes blood sugar. While on the fertility diet, you will look for whole-grain carbohydrates. These foods include all three edible parts of the grain: the bran, endosperm, and germ. These have never been removed, altered, processed or re-added to the foods from which they first came (as is often the case with industrially produced whole-grain bread (see page 43).

Slow Carbs

While you are trying to achieve conception, carbohydrates must be part of your diet. Brain cells, in particular, need a ready supply of fuel. Keep in mind that it is not the amount of carbohydrates in the diet that affects fertility (and overall health), it is the type of carbohydrates. Good carbohydrates, and the slow, steady release of glucose they offer the brain and fertility system, have been positively linked with higher ovulation rates and increased pregnancy rates.

The Glycemic Index

A few words about wheat, the glycemic index, and high glycemic foods: Women in the Nurses' Health Study who consumed carbohydrates and other foods with the highest glycemic load were 92 percent more likely to have experienced ovulatory infertility than women who ate a diet with a low glycemic load. Because the participants in the Nurses' Health Study filled out questionnaires about what carbohydrates were in their daily diet, a great deal of information about the type of carbohydrates consumed and their impact on fertility was gathered. In general, cold breakfast cereals (even those fortified with essential fertility nutrients), white rice, and potatoes were positively linked with a higher risk of ovulatory infertility. Slow carbs were linked with a lower risk.

Wheat in its most refined forms, including most commercially produced baked goods, increases blood sugar more rapidly than do other refined carbohydrates, such as potato chips. This has to do with the carbohydrate structure of these foods and how our digestive system converts the carbohydrates in wheat to glucose. The carbohydrates in wheat are 75 percent amylopectin A and 25 percent amylose. Our bodies easily digest the amylopectin A and rapidly convert it to glucose. (Amylose is less efficiently digested.)

A comparative look at the impact of carbohydrates on blood sugar was first done in 1981, when a study at the University of Toronto launched the concept of the glycemic index (GI). Specifically, the higher the blood sugar after consuming a specific food, as compared with glucose, the higher the GI. In that study, the GI of white bread was 69 while the GI of whole grain bread was 72. Sucrose (table sugar) was 59. It is the body's ease of digesting the amylopectin A that gives bread made from wheat a higher GI than that of table sugar.

The glycemic indexes of hundreds of foods have been measured since that first study. Generally speaking, a food with a GI of 55 or less is considered a low GI food. These foods have a slow, steady effect on blood sugar and insulin. Medium glycemic foods measure between 56 and 69, while high GI foods measure above 70. Whole-grain bread, whose healthful benefits have been touted by many in the health-care industry, can be perilous to your overall health.

Gluten-Free Grains

The type of wheat you choose can have a significant impact on your wellness and fertility. Choose carbohydrates that are made from gluten-free grains, such as quinoa and brown rice, or unadulterated forms of wheat, such as whole spelt or farro—wheat's ancient cousins—and limit foods made from modern wheat strains, such as durum wheat.

Gluten is a protein composite made of a gliadin and a glutenin, which are found in foods made from wheat and related grain species, such as barley and rye. Avoiding gluten may help you return to fertility, particularly if you have problems digesting it. Celiac disease, a serious digestive disorder in which the immune system responds to ingested gluten by attacking the intestinal wall, is estimated to be responsible for up to 8 percent of all cases of unexplained infertility. Celiac disease and other issues related to digestive health can limit your body's ability to properly absorb nutrients, a serious issue for general wellness and especially for women trying to conceive. Over time, in consultation with your health-care provider, you may want to eliminate gluten-bearing grains from your diet entirely.

Smart Slow Carbs—Eat These Often

Smart slow carbs, or whole-grain carbohydrates with a low GI, include the following foods (the per serving GI is in parentheses):

- Brown and wild rice (55)
- Whole or flaked quinoa; the germ, endosperm, and bran are still included (35)
- Whole or rolled oats (58)
- Bulgur (46), spelt (45), farro (40), and other forms of ancient wheat
- Legumes such as black-eyed peas (42), black beans (30), navy beans (38), and lentils (29)

Spiky Carbs—Eat These Rarely

Spiky carbs, or carbohydrates that convert efficiently to glucose, include the following:

- Soft drinks (68)
- White pasta (61)
- White rice (64)
- Baking potato (85)
- White bread (69), multigrain bread (72), and whole-wheat bread (72) made from modern wheat
- Pizza (80)
- Frozen bagels (72)
- Cakes and tarts (65+)
- Pastries: cheese danish (59)
- Doughnuts (76)

For overall wellness and fertility-positive eating, try not to focus on specific GI numbers. What matters is the big picture. You do not have to give up pasta and cereal, but you may want to change the type of pasta and cereal you eat, especially if they are currently a regular part of your diet. Whole-grain pasta is better than white pasta, for example. Flip over the box and read the nutrition facts panel. Take a close look at the numbers for total carbohydrates, fiber, and protein. Most nutritionists believe that at least 5 grams of fiber and 4 grams of protein per serving are best for satiety (how long you feel full after eating), as well as for counteracting the quick rush of sugar to the bloodstream from spiky carbs.

If you do choose to eat bread, try to get a loaf that delivers close to 5 grams of fiber and 4 grams of protein per serving, and you are off to a good start on your new eating plan. Of course, some packaged goods manufacturers boost the nutrition facts with fillers such as whey (a by-product of cheese making). The goal is to choose products that naturally contain whole nutrition, not products artificially boosted to look whole. If in doubt, read the ingredients list. Whole foods have very short ingredient lists and include minimally processed ingredients, such as whole oats or whole buckwheat. These whole ingredients should be listed first.

Other Slow Carbohydrates

Carbohydrates come from other foods in addition to grains and beans. Whole fruits, vegetables, and nuts are also considered carbohydrates, and almost all of these, when consumed in their whole form, are low on the glycemic index scale. Of course, the big exception is white potato (85 for one).

Adding some fat to your slow carbs helps slow down the digestion of carbohydrates and boosts satiety. Remember, you are not worried about quantity, you are worried about quality.

Fats

All humans need fats for optimum health. Our bodies use fats for energy, to protect nerve cells, turn genes on and off, rev up or calm inflammation, and countless other functions. Regarding fertility, fats enable us to absorb vitamin D and protect sex hormones, among other functions.

Of course, fat also gets a bad rap for some of the negative consequences associated with eating too much of the wrong types. Too much cholesterol from saturated fat can harm the circulatory system and lead to numerous other problems. When attempting to conceive, you need to eat fats—more of the healthful ones and fewer of the rest.

Saturated Fats and Trans Fats

Saturated fats come mostly from animal products. These fats, which are high in cholesterol, are linked with heart and circulatory problems, insulin resistance, and endometriosis. You do need some cholesterol in your diet to support fertility, since your body uses cholesterol to make hormones, including progesterone and testosterone. When you are trying to get pregnant, a daily serving of whole milk or another full-fat dairy food can help you fight ovulatory infertility, and is considered a healthful part of the fertility diet.

Trans-fatty acids (TFAs) are found in small amounts in various animal products, such as beef, pork, lamb, and the butterfat in butter and milk. TFAs are also formed during the process of hydrogenation. They increase harmful low-density lipoproteins LDL in your body ("bad cholesterol") and decrease protective high-density lipoproteins HDL ("good cholesterol").

In a large long-term study conducted by the Harvard School of Public Health and Harvard Medical School, a positive link was found between trans fats and ovulatory infertility. Women who ate as little as 4 grams of trans fats per day were 70 percent less likely to become pregnant. Trans fats interfere with ovulatory function, cause or exacerbate insulin resistance, and interfere with hormone production and balance. Trans fats do not have a place in the fertility diet.

In packaged foods and fast food, TFAs offer a shelf-stable source of fat. After packaged food producers were legally required to list trans fats in the nutrition facts box on each package, many removed some or all of the TFAs from their products. In most cases, the TFAs were swapped for saturated fat. Read labels carefully on all packaged foods, including crackers, bread, and baked goods, as these products are often a hidden source of saturated fat.

In that same Harvard study, saturated fat in red meat also appeared to obstruct fertility. In fact, ovulatory infertility was 39 percent more likely to occur in women with the highest intake of animal protein than in women with the lowest intake. Women with the highest intake of plant-based protein were least likely to experience ovulatory infertility. The study led researchers to conclude that replacing carbohydrates with animal protein boosted the risk of ovulatory infertility by 20 percent. On the other hand, replacing carbs with plant-based proteins reduced the risk of ovulatory infertility by 43 percent. And finally, replacing animal proteins with plant-based proteins lowered the risk of ovulatory infertility by 50 percent. In sum: Eat more protein from plants.

Eating out can be a minefield of saturated and trans fat foods. Many restaurants, especially—but not exclusively—fast-food chains, still use trans fat in the form of partially hydrogenated oil to make fried foods. Get picky about what types of foods you choose when eating out. Ask lots of questions. Do not be afraid to eat some saturated fats, but do avoid trans fats.

The fertility diet does not suggest giving up animal proteins. But flexibility when selecting protein is key to a fertility-positive lifestyle. Put a smaller piece of meat on your plate. Then surround it with healthful carbohydrates from a variety of sources. And be sure to fill your cup once a day with whole milk.

Unsaturated Fats

Derived mainly from plants, unsaturated fats are essential for optimum wellness and fertility. These fats are liquid at room temperature, in the form of oil. Most cooking oils contain a combination of monounsaturated and polyunsaturated fats. Olive oil, canola oil, and peanut oil are all high in monosaturated fat, which lowers harmful LDL cholesterol and boosts protective HDL cholesterol. Monosaturated fat also eases inflammation and heighten the body's sensitivity to insulin.

Polyunsaturated fat is found in safflower oil, soybean oil, corn oil, sesame oil, and flaxseed oil. This type of unsaturated fat is part of the omega-3 and omega-6 family (for more information on omega-3 and omega-6 fatty acids, see page 36). Like monounsaturated fats, polyunsaturated fat lowers harmful LDL cholesterol and boosts protective HDL cholesterol.

Smart Fats

Smart fats are whole fats. They are mostly unsaturated. Eat plenty of these, but don't forget the daily portion of full-fat dairy.

- Fatty fish, such as wild salmon, herring, sardines, blue fish, and mackerel
- Nuts and seeds, such as almonds, cashews, flax, hemp, pine nuts, pumpkin, pistachios, and walnuts
- Grass-fed beef
- Oils rich in omega-3 and omega-6 fatty acids, such as olive, canola, flaxseed, grapeseed, hemp, and pumpkin seed
- Eggs

A Word About Dairy Products

In the Harvard study described on page 44, total dairy intake did little to influence fertility. What did make the difference was the type of dairy products. The more low-fat dairy in a woman's diet, the more likely she was to have had trouble getting pregnant. Conversely, the more full-fat dairy products in a woman's diet, the less likely she was to have had trouble. One half-cup serving a day of products made from whole milk was found to tip the scale in favor of fertility.

The hormones that occur naturally in whole milk have a great impact on fertility. The milk we drink today is richer in hormones than the milk people drank a century ago. Today's milk includes an abundance of female and male hormones, such as prolactin, estrogen, testosterone, and progesterone. One reason for this change is that our milk comes from cows that are often pregnant, whereas a century ago dairy cows were milked when they were in the early stages of pregnancy, if they were pregnant at all. When milk is skimmed, these hormones are removed with the cream. A few hormones are left behind, including prolactin, which is important for breast-feeding. The study's researchers concluded that drinking milk can affect the balance of sex hormones. Products that contain whole milk or the cream skimmed from whole milk contain enough hormones to affect the ovaries and other tissues.

Smart Full-Fat Dairy

Full-fat dairy products should be consumed in moderation, one to two half-cup servings a day is optimal. Smart full-fat dairy includes the following:

- Milk
- Ice cream
- Cheese

Advice for the Lactose Intolerant

If you have difficulty digesting milk-based products or you simply don't enjoy them, it is neither necessary nor recommended that you force yourself to eat these foods. Whether it supports fertility or not, food should be joyful, not harmful or unpleasant. A serving of full-fat dairy is just one dietary option out of a whole range of lifestyle choices that are fertility positive.

Protein

Every cell in the body contains protein. It is one of the building blocks of life. The amino acids in the body's protein helps in the development of egg production and sperm maturation, as well as in the production of hormones. Our bodies break down the protein we eat and use it to build up new protein. Foods with protein are a must for any diet, including the fertility diet. Once again, the amount and type of protein you choose is key to improving fertility.

As noted earlier, the large long-term study conducted by the Harvard School of Public Health and Harvard Medical School concluded that reducing animal protein intake while increasing vegetable protein intake, such as beans, peas, soybeans, or any sort of nut, resulted in modest protection against ovulatory infertility. Moreover, eating most of your daily protein from plant sources reduces the risk of heart disease, stroke, and other cardiovascular problems.

The Iron Question

In the Harvard Study, women who got most of their iron from meat (heme iron) were not protected from ovulatory infertility. Woman who got most of their iron from fruits, vegetables, beans, and supplements (nonheme iron), improved their chances of getting pregnant.

A Word about Fish and Mercury

As noted earlier, fish and other seafood are excellent sources of protein, but they may contain mercury, an industrial contaminant. Women who wish to conceive, as well as pregnant and nursing women and the parents of small children, should take care when selecting and eating fish and shellfish (see page 36–37 for more information). While king mackerel contains high levels of mercury, there is no mercury advisory for Atlantic mackerel, a species with one of the highest levels of beneficial omega-3 fatty acids, in addition to protein. Two or three 6-ounce portions of fish per week are recommended.

In general, the smaller the fish, the lower the risk of accumulated mercury in its flesh. In addition to Atlantic mackerel, some safe choices for the fertility diet when eaten in moderation are bluefish, halibut, herring, oysters, salmon, sardines, shrimp, and trout.

Sea vegetables and seaweed are also high in omega-3 fatty acids. Sprinkle a bit of nori, kombu, or dulse over soup or rice.

Smart Protein

Smart protein is mostly plant-based, but not exclusively. A good approach is a flexitarian one—some protein from vegetables each day, and a smaller amount from animals. Use as many different sources as you can. Get cozy with your grocer or local farmers' market. Find out what is in season, because seasonal foods are at their peak nutritive value and have been shipped shorter distances, which means they have been harvested when more ripe and flavorful. Good sources of protein include the following:

- Carob
- Eggs
- Full-fat dairy
- Lean meats, including leaner cuts of grass-fed beef, buffalo, chicken, lamb, pork, and turkey
- Legumes, such as beans of any color (black, white, navy, pinto), black-eyed peas, lentils, and soybeans
- Nuts, such as almonds, pecans, pignoli (pine nuts), pistachios, and walnuts; nut butters such as almond, hazelnut, and peanut
- Shellfish, including crab, mussels, oysters, and shrimp
- Wild, fatty fish, such as Atlantic mackerel, herring, and salmon

Beverages

Drinking enough liquids to replenish what is lost during the day matters for overall wellness and is just as important for the fertility diet. How much you need depends on how active you are and the temperature and humidity outside. Generally speaking, we all need about 8 cups of liquid every day.

Caffeinated Drinks

There is no consensus on the safety of caffeinated beverages for women who want to conceive (or already have). Some research implicates caffeine for higher rates of birth defects; other research denies the caffeine connection. With regard to fertility, in the study conducted by the Harvard School of Public Health of more than eighteen thousand female nurses, researchers concluded that caffeine had no impact on ovulation, but it is possible that caffeine can make it more difficult for the fallopian tubes to contract and relax, slowing the movement of a fertilized egg to the uterus. Caffeine may also make the lining of the uterus less hospitable to a fertilized egg.

Research done as part of another study at Harvard, described earlier in this chapter, found that caffeine ingested from soda negatively affected overall fertility while the caffeine ingested from coffee or tea had no impact on fertility. Could it be the sugar? The average can of soda contains 3 tablespoons plus 1 teaspoon of sugar (often in the form of corn syrup, cane syrup, or molasses). The body digests sugar immediately and as a result, blood sugar and insulin levels spike, which affects fertility. As we discussed earlier on page 39–44, minimizing this rise and fall of blood sugar is task one for our overall health and a fertility-positive diet.

To be more fertility positive, drink caffeinated coffee or tea in moderation. Limit yourself to no more than two or three 8-ounce cups of coffee; you can get away with drinking more tea. (A home-brewed 8-ounce cup of coffee contains between 90 and 120 milligrams of caffeine.) And if you really want to be safe, consider giving up caffeine altogether.

It can be hard to make a big change to your diet, and giving up caffeine is no exception. Coffee drinkers may want to switch to a blend of caffeinated and decaffeinated coffee before giving up caffeinated coffee. Switching to black tea, which delivers roughly half of the caffeine of an equivalent amount of coffee, can be a good intermediate step. If you are giving up soda, unsweetened fruit-flavored water can provide a intermediate step away from sweetened carbonated beverages before giving them up for good.

Alcoholic Drinks

As with caffeine, there are many uncertainties surrounding the connection between alcohol and fertility. Keep in mind that alcohol has no positive impact on fertility (jokes aside!), so you are not missing anything by giving it up. If you do want to drink while trying to conceive, limit drinking to the days when you are menstruating or preovulatory. To improve your overall fertility, eliminate alcohol entirely.

THE BIG PICTURE

To visualize the fertility diet, make a drawing: First, draw a circle near the center-bottom of the paper. This is the typical 10-inch kitchen plate. Think of what you put on your plate at breakfast, lunch, and dinner. Divide the plate into four sections, one of them slightly larger than the rest. Color the largest section green for vegetables, and another section red or purple for fruits. Add a blue section for protein, and a brown section for whole carbs. This is a good visual reminder that the more veggies you put on your plate, the better. Place a variety of foods on your plate in each category, and make sure you have enough fats. The foods should be ones that satisfy you and provide maximum nutrition. Make sure you cover breakfast, lunch, and dinner.

Now, put a few things next to your plate: Draw an 8-ounce water glass to represent liquids. You can add a separate glass or small bowl for the daily serving of whole milk or ice cream. To represent other fats, place a small oil decanter next to the water glass. Then draw a small yellow tablet near the water glass; this is your multivitamin.

Put your drawing on a clipboard or in a folder with your daily fertility chart, or in another place (like the refrigerator door) where you will see it frequently. It will encourage you to make whole foods, healthful fats, and whole fruits and vegetables the foundation of your daily eating plan.

What to Stock in Your Pantry

- Beans and legumes such as chickpeas (garbanzo beans), black beans, cannellini beans, lentils, and split peas
- Gluten-free whole grains that are minimally processed, such as brown rice, buckwheat, oats, and quinoa

- Heritage varieties of gluten-bearing grains, minimally processed, such as farro, rye, and spelt
- Plant-based oils, such as canola, grapeseed, and olive
- Dried seaweed and sea vegetables, such as dulse and nori
- Nuts such as almonds, hazelnuts, and walnuts —whole, or as milks or oils
- Seeds such as chia, flax, hemp, and sesame—whole, or as milks or oils
- Canned or vacuum-packed fish, such as anchovies, wild salmon, and sardines
- Dark chocolate
- Green tea

What to Keep in Your Freezer or Refrigerator

- Eggs
- Fish, including anchovies, herring, Atlantic mackerel, sardines, trout, and wild Alaskan salmon
- Fruits (organic whenever possible), including apples, berries (strawberry, blueberry, blackberry), figs, pears, limes, lemons, and stone fruits (apricot, cherry, peach, plum)
- Lean meats, including leaner cuts of grass-fed beef, buffalo, chicken, lamb, pork, and turkey
- Full-fat cheese and whole milk
- Organic soybeans in the form of tofu or whole beans (edamame)
- Shellfish, including crab, mussels, oysters, and shrimp
- Vegetables (organic whenever possible), including avocado, celery, cucumbers, green beans, root vegetables (carrots, parsnips, turnips, rutabaga), squash, sweet potato, and tomato
- All of the dark green leafy vegetables (cabbage, collard greens, kale, turnip greens)

Ten Steps Toward Conception Using the Fertility Diet

1. Start taking a daily prenatal vitamin about three months before you want to begin trying to become pregnant. Ask your partner to begin taking a multivitamin.

2. Include one to two servings of whole milk, full-fat ice cream, or full-fat cheese in your daily diet.
3. Reduce the amount of caffeine you drink, or eliminate it entirely.
4. Limit the alcohol you drink to the days when you are menstruating or preovulatory, or eliminate it entirely.
5. Eliminate caffeinated sugary sodas from your diet entirely.
6. Eat a wide variety of foods, including proteins, carbohydrates, and fats.
7. When selecting proteins, aim for 50 percent or more of the day's proteins to come from vegetable sources.
8. When selecting animal proteins, choose lean cuts.
9. Add more whole-grain, gluten-free carbohydrates to your diet.
10. Reduce or eliminate white sugar from your diet (but the occasional piece of dark chocolate is encouraged!).

CHAPTER FOUR

7-Day Meal Plan

Just the thought of a meal plan makes some of us anxious. You may have been down the diet road more times than you care to count. The fertility diet meal plan is really just a guideline, though, to encourage you to make good dietary choices. Fertility is the main goal. One of the underlying principles of the plan is that you will *want* to eat healthful food if it tastes good.

HOW TO USE THIS MEAL PLAN

Many of us do not spend a lot of time cooking these days, for one reason or another. But cooking your food is the only way to know *exactly* what you are eating. Restaurants and the take-out foods in supermarkets are notorious for adding salt, fats, and other flavor enhancers. If you absolutely cannot cook, by all means choose premade foods that follow the fertility diet guidelines. (Read pages 34–36 for the list of foods that include important nutrients for fertility.) Remember, anytime that you spend cooking and preparing your own food is a step in the right direction, a step toward fertility and good health.

The fertility diet meal plan includes a daily balanced mix of protein, carbohydrates, and fats. Three complete meals are included each day as well as two snacks. The rough caloric goal is 2,000 calories per day. You can choose what time of day you need your snacks and pretty much everything else. If you do not like the vegetable, fruit, or grain choice we suggest in a recipe, substitute another one. Food should be fun, shared with loved ones and friends. Food should be joyful and nourishing. Food supports life. *Santé!*

MONDAY

Breakfast
Hot Quinoa Breakfast Cereal with Fruit and Flax

Lunch
Tofu Slaw with Sesame-Tamari Dressing

Snack
Cup of full-fat ice cream

Dinner
Mackerel and Lentil Salad

Snack
Purchased hummus with rice crackers

TUESDAY

Breakfast
Baked Apples with Almonds and Honey

Lunch
Cream of Tomato Soup with flax crackers

Snack
Purchased guacamole and tortilla chips

Dinner
Purchased rotisserie chicken with Roasted Balsamic Brussels
    Sprouts with Pignoli

Snack
Kale chips

WEDNESDAY

Breakfast
Rolled oats with sliced pears and blue cheese

Lunch
Purchased black bean dip with yucca or tortilla chips

Snack

Gluten-free granola

Dinner

Yellow Dal with Split Peas

Snack

Purchased pumpernickel bagel (only eat half) with cream cheese

THURSDAY

Breakfast

Winter Smoothie

Lunch

Spinach Salad with Toasted Walnuts and Walnut Oil Dressing

Snack

Purchased muhammara (walnut red-pepper dip) and pretzel sticks

Dinner

Old-Fashioned Stuffed Peppers

Snack

Hazelnut Butter and Banana Sandwich

FRIDAY

Breakfast

Whole-milk cheese breakfast with wheat-free granola and fruit

Lunch

Rice and Lentil Salad

Snack

Peanut butter and honey sandwich

Dinner

Citrus-Soy Salmon with Coconut Ginger Rice

Snack

Roasted Mixed Nuts with Tamari

SATURDAY

Breakfast
Breakfast Burrito

Lunch
Cannellini Bean Salad with Mint and Parsley topped with purchased olive oil–packed tuna

Snack
Purchased toasted, seasoned garbanzo beans

Dinner
Buffalo Burgers with Smoky Flavors

Snack
Full-fat ice cream

SUNDAY

Breakfast
Purchased cheese blintzes with fresh fruit

Lunch
Tomato Bean Soup with Farro

Snack
Grape-seed-oil-popped popcorn

Dinner
Grilled Bluefish

Snack
Dark Chocolate Nut Clusters

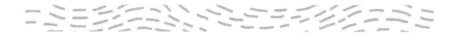

PART TWO

Recipes

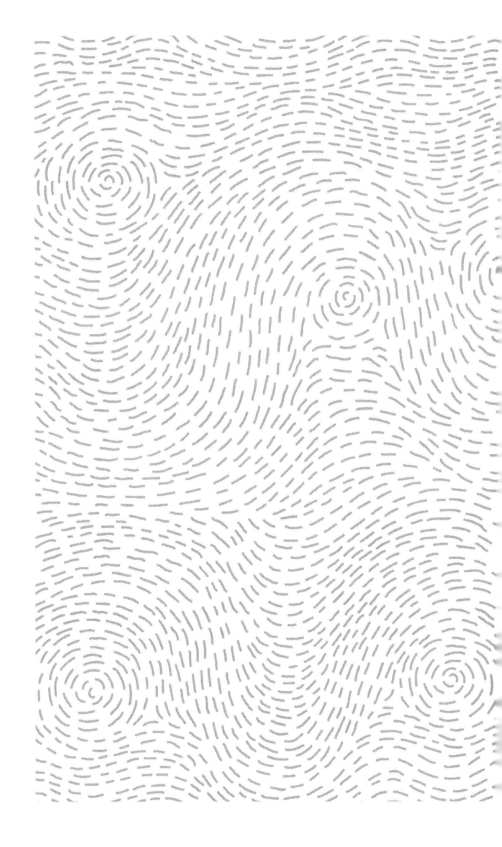

Snacks

DARK CHOCOLATE NUT CLUSTERS

ROASTED MIXED NUTS WITH TAMARI

HAZELNUT BUTTER AND BANANA SANDWICH

GLUTEN-FREE GRANOLA

KALE CHIPS

Breakfast

HOT QUINOA BREAKFAST CEREAL WITH FRUIT AND FLAX

BREAKFAST BURRITO

RICOTTA WITH WHEAT-FREE GRANOLA AND FRUIT

BAKED APPLES WITH ALMONDS AND HONEY

WINTER SMOOTHIE

Lunch

TOFU SLAW WITH SESAME-TAMARI DRESSING

SPINACH SALAD WITH TOASTED WALNUTS AND WALNUT OIL DRESSING

RICE AND LENTIL SALAD

CANNELLINI BEAN SALAD WITH MINT AND PARSLEY

CREAM OF TOMATO SOUP

TOMATO BEAN SOUP WITH FARRO

Dinner

BUFFALO BURGERS WITH SMOKY FLAVORS

CITRUS-SOY SALMON

continued ▶

DINNER *continued* ▶

COCONUT GINGER RICE

YELLOW DAL WITH SPLIT PEAS

ROASTED BALSAMIC BRUSSELS SPROUTS WITH PIGNOLI

OLD-FASHIONED STUFFED PEPPERS

SALMON POKE

MACKEREL AND LENTIL SALAD

GRILLED BLUEFISH

Snacks

Dark Chocolate Nut Clusters

MAKES 4½ DOZEN

▶ CALORIES 191.6, FAT 15 G, CHOLESTEROL 4 MG, SODIUM 11 MG,
CARBOHYDRATES 19 G, FIBER 3 G, PROTEIN 2 G, IRON 9%, FOLIC ACID 0.2%

*This is a great recipe for getting your chocolate without spiking your blood
sugar. And chocolate gives you a boost of beneficial flavonoids.*

1 CUP PLUS 3 TABLESPOONS (9 OUNCES) MELTED DARK
    CHOCOLATE, 70% COCOA
1½ CUPS WHOLE ALMONDS
COARSE OR LAVENDER SEA SALT

1. Line a baking sheet with parchment paper or a baking mat.

2. Place 1 teaspoon of the melted chocolate on the paper and top with
6 almonds. Drizzle the almonds with 1 tablespoon of melted chocolate.
Repeat the process with the remaining almonds and chocolate.

3. Sprinkle the clusters with sea salt, and refrigerate until firm.

Roasted Mixed Nuts with Tamari

MAKES ABOUT 6 ONE-CUP SERVINGS

▶ CALORIES 207, FAT 14.6 G, CHOLESTEROL 0 MG, SODIUM 540.8 MG, CARBOHYDRATES 13.5 G, FIBER 2.8 G, PROTEIN 6.7 G, IRON 1.6%, FOLIC ACID .5%

If you enjoy grazing on those snacks of mixed cereals and pretzels, this will be right up your alley. When cool, pack it in portion-size containers to take to work or the gym.

COCONUT OIL OR CANOLA OIL FOR THE BAKING SHEETS
8 OUNCES PEANUTS
8 OUNCES CASHEWS
8 OUNCES ALMONDS
4 OUNCES PUMPKIN SEEDS
4 OUNCES HAZELNUTS
½ CUP WHEAT-FREE TAMARI
2 CUPS UNSALTED POPCORN
½ CUP UNSWEETENED COCONUT FLAKES

1. Preheat the oven to 275°F.

2. Lightly grease two baking sheets with coconut oil.

3. Combine the nuts and seeds in a large bowl. Add the tamari and toss to coat.

4. Allow to soak for 10 minutes; then spread out evenly on the baking sheets.

5. Bake for 20 to 25 minutes. Cool completely on the baking sheet. Transfer to a large bowl, toss with the popcorn and coconut, and serve.

Hazelnut Butter and Banana Sandwich

SERVES 1

▶ CALORIES 321, FAT 6.6 G, CHOLESTEROL 0 MG, SODIUM 195.8 MG, CARBOHYDRATES 62 G, FIBER 6.5 G, PROTEIN 5.5 G, IRON 6%, FOLIC ACID 0%

For some folks, this simple sandwich is breakfast. Since the ingredients are portable, it also makes a satisfying afternoon snack on the go.

1 SLICE SPELT OR MILLET BREAD

1 TABLESPOON SUGAR-FREE HAZELNUT AND CHOCOLATE SPREAD OR ROASTED HAZELNUT SPREAD

2 TABLESPOON SLICED BANANAS

1. Spread the bread with the hazelnut and chocolate mixture.

2. Top with the banana slices.

Gluten-Free Granola

▶ CALORIES 184.8, FAT 7 G, CHOLESTEROL 0 MG, SODIUM 5.1 MG, CARBOHYDRATES 27.4 G, FIBER 3.5 G, PROTEIN 4.3 G, IRON 7.9%, FOLIC ACID 1.1%

Rolled oats are digested slowly, and the walnut oil adds a nice richness. If you like, add a tablespoon of crushed flaxseed or flaxseed oil to the oats when you add the fruit and nuts —this boosts your essential fatty acids. You can also use the granola as a topping for ice cream.

4 CUPS ROLLED OATS
⅓ CUP HONEY
¼ CUP WALNUT OIL
2 TEASPOONS VANILLA EXTRACT
1 TEASPOON GROUND CINNAMON
1 CUP MIXED DRIED FRUIT
1 CUP CHOPPED, TOASTED MIXED NUTS OR SEEDS, SUCH AS
    WALNUTS, CASHEWS, PECANS, AND SUNFLOWER SEEDS

1. Preheat the oven to 300°F.

2. In a large bowl, combine the oats, honey, oil, vanilla, and cinnamon. Spread out evenly on a large rimmed baking sheet.

3. Bake for 15 minutes. Stir the oats well and bake for another 15 minutes, or until evenly toasted. Let cool to room temperature.

4. Transfer the granola to a large bowl; add the fruit and nuts, and stir thoroughly to combine. Serve immediately or store in an airtight container for up to 2 weeks.

64   Fertility *for Beginners*

Kale Chips

▶   CALORIES 70, FAT 7.1 G, CHOLESTEROL 0 MG, SODIUM 8.8 MG, CARBOHYDRATES 2 G, FIBER .5 G, PROTEIN .8 G, IRON 2%, FOLIC ACID 0%

If you're looking for a crunchy snack to munch on instead of potato chips, you'll love these kale chips. Feeling lazy? Instead of tearing up the kale leaves, you can roast them whole. The stems are quite chewy.

2 HEADS CURLY LEAF KALE, LEAVES SEPARATED
2 TABLESPOONS EXTRA-VIRGIN OLIVE OIL
PINCH OF SEA SALT

1. Preheat the oven to 325°F.

2. Tear the kale into bite-size pieces, removing any tough stems. Transfer to a medium bowl and add the olive oil.

3. Using your hands, gently massage the olive oil into the kale. Spread out the kale on a baking sheet in a single layer and sprinkle with the sea salt.

4. Bake for 10 to 15 minutes, or until crispy. Serve immediately, or cool and store in an airtight container.

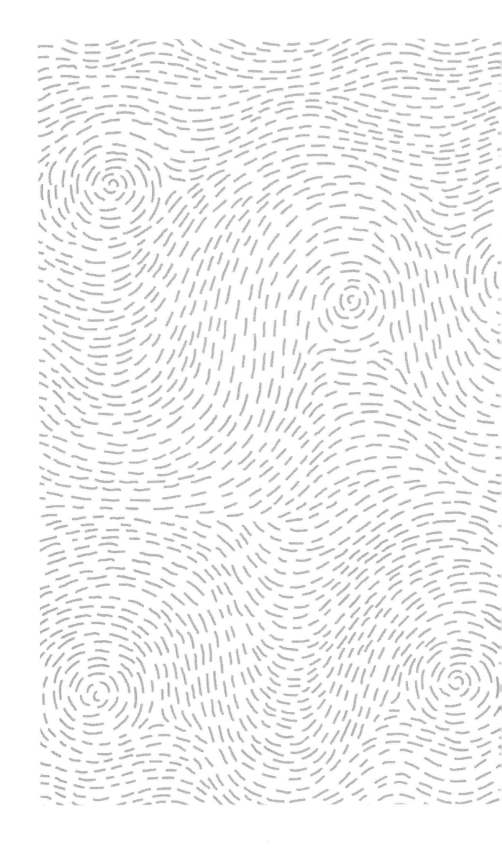

Breakfast

Hot Quinoa Breakfast Cereal with Fruit and Flax

SERVES 4

▶ CALORIES 341, FAT 13.8 G, CHOLESTEROL 0.0 MG, SODIUM 0.0 MG, CARBOHYDRATES 48 G, FIBER 6 G, PROTEIN 8 G, IRON 24%, FOLIC ACID 3%

For such a tiny seed, quinoa contains an ideal combination of protein, fiber, and fat to keep you energized and satisfied throughout the morning. To save time, you can use flaked quinoa. It contains the endosperm and the bran, and provides the same nutritional benefits as whole-grain quinoa but cooks in just under one minute in boiling water. If using flaked quinoa, after bringing the water to a boil, add the quinoa, apricots, and salt. Stir, remove from the heat, and let rest for one minute before proceeding with step 2.

2 CUPS FILTERED WATER

1 CUP WHOLE-GRAIN QUINOA

¼ CUP DRIED APRICOTS, DICED

PINCH OF SEA SALT

1 TABLESPOON DRIED BLUEBERRIES (OR FRESH IF IN SEASON)

½ TEASPOON GROUND CINNAMON

⅛ TEASPOON GROUND NUTMEG

1 TABLESPOON FLAXSEED OIL OR ALMOND OIL

1. In a medium saucepan, bring the water to a rolling boil. Add the quinoa, apricots, and salt. Return the water to a boil, lower the heat, and simmer gently, covered, for about 20 minutes, or until the water is completely absorbed. Remove from the heat.

2. Stir in the blueberries and allow the cereal to rest for 5 minutes.

3. Stir in the cinnamon, nutmeg, and oil. Taste and adjust the seasonings as needed.

Breakfast Burrito

SERVES 2

▶ CALORIES 389, FAT 29 G, CHOLESTEROL 231 MG, SODIUM 473 MG, CARBOHYDRATES 15.9 G, FIBER 2.8 G, PROTEIN 18 G, IRON 10.4%, FOLIC ACID 15.9%

This classic dish is ideal for improving fertility because it is chock-full of iron, whole milk fat, and B vitamins, including a healthy dose of folic acid.

2 CORN TORTILLAS
1 TABLESPOON EXTRA-VIRGIN OLIVE OIL
2 EGGS
2 TABLESPOONS SHREDDED CHEDDAR CHEESE
2 SLICES REDUCED-FAT TURKEY BACON, COOKED AND CHOPPED
1 TABLESPOON SALSA
½ AVOCADO, SLICED

1. Place the tortillas in a large nonstick skillet and warm gently over low heat, turning once. Transfer to plate.

2. Meanwhile, heat the olive oil in another nonstick skillet over medium heat. Add the eggs and cook, stirring often, until cooked through, about 2 minutes. Divide the scrambled eggs between the tacos. Top with the cheese, bacon, salsa, and avocado, and serve immediately.

Ricotta with Wheat-Free Granola and Fruit

SERVES 2

▶ CALORIES 400, FAT 23 G, CHOLESTEROL 62 MG, SODIUM 113 MG, CARBOHYDRATES 32.1 G, FIBER 3.7 G, PROTEIN 9.6 G, IRON 10.2%, FOLIC ACID 10%

Locally sourced honey is said to provide a boost to the immune system and relief from seasonal allergies. In winter, substitute dried fruit for fresh.

1 CUP WHOLE-MILK RICOTTA
½ TEASPOON GRATED LEMON ZEST
2 TABLESPOONS GLUTEN-FREE GRANOLA, HOMEMADE (PAGE 64)
    OR STORE-BOUGHT
2 TABLESPOONS SLICED SEASONAL FRUIT
1 TEASPOON LOCAL HONEY

1. In a small bowl, whisk together the ricotta and lemon zest. Let rest for a few minutes.

2. Top with the granola, fruit, and a drizzle of honey.

Baked Apples with Almonds and Honey

SERVES 4

▶ CALORIES 170, FAT 6.5 G, CHOLESTEROL 11 MG, SODIUM 1 MG, CARBOHYDRATES 26 G, FIBER 4 G, PROTEIN 1.6 G, IRON 2%, FOLIC ACID 0%

This homey recipe is best in fall, when apples are at their peak. Almost any fill-ing works with apples, so try sweet and savory fruits, vegetables, and nuts until you find a mix that hits the spot. If you like, you can make these the night before and refrigerate. Bring to room temperature or warm gently before serving.

4 CORTLAND APPLES (OR OTHER BAKING APPLES)
4 TEASPOONS SLICED ALMONDS
4 TEASPOONS DRIED CRANBERRIES
4 TEASPOONS HONEY
1½ TABLESPOONS BUTTER, CUT INTO 4 PIECES
½ CUP UNFILTERED APPLE CIDER
1 TEASPOON ALMOND OIL

1. Preheat the oven to 400°F.

2. Using a melon baller, scoop out the seeds and core of each apple, leaving about ½ inch at the bottom of the apple intact.

3. Place the apples in a baking dish and stuff each with 1 teaspoon of the almonds and 1 teaspoon of the cranberries. Top with 1 teaspoon of honey and 1 teaspoon (one piece) of butter.

4. Add the apple cider to the baking dish and bake the apples, basting every 5 to 7 minutes, until tender, 25 to 35 minutes. Serve immediately or cool and refrigerate to serve later.

Winter Smoothie

SERVES 2

▶ CALORIES 291, FAT 11.1 G, CHOLESTEROL 0 MG, SODIUM 143 MG, CARBOHYDRATES 48.9 G, FIBER 10.7 G, PROTEIN 6 G, IRON 19%, FOLIC ACID 18.5%

Hiding spinach in a smoothie makes it taste so good you will not even notice it is there. If you like, substitute ¼ cup of unsweetened whole-milk Greek yogurt for the avocado.

1 CUP ALMOND MILK

3 CUPS TORN KALE OR SPINACH LEAVES

1 BANANA, PEELED

1 ORANGE, PEELED

1 SMALL GREEN APPLE, CORED AND ROUGHLY CHOPPED

1 CUP FROZEN PEACHES

1 AVOCADO, PEELED AND PITTED

Combine the ingredients in a blender in the order listed and blend on high speed until smooth. Serve and enjoy.

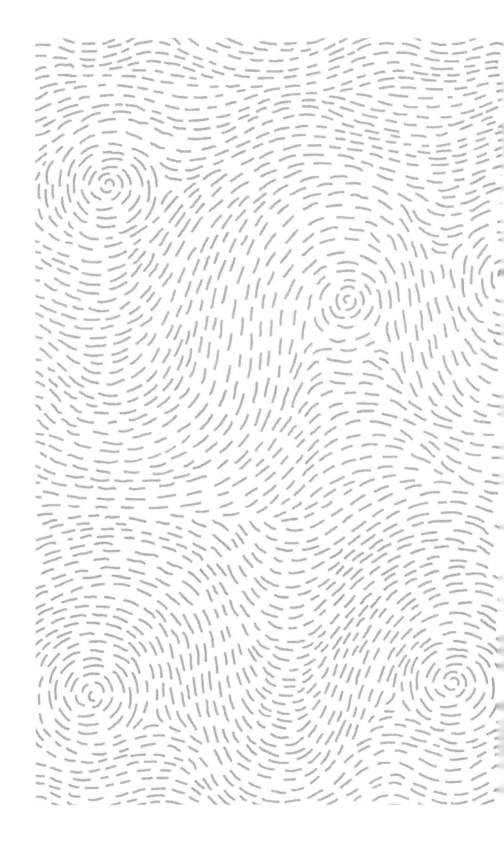

Lunch

Tofu Slaw with Sesame-Tamari Dressing

SERVES 4

▶ CALORIES 602, FAT 52.9 G, CHOLESTEROL 0 MG, SODIUM 785 MG, CARBOHYDRATES 22.2 G, FIBER 7.3 G, PROTEIN 17.3 G, IRON 39.5%, FOLIC ACID 31.3%

Tofu gives this salad a boost of soy isoflavones, a valuable nutrient. If your ob-gyn or nutritionist recommends a soy-free diet, roasted chicken or cooked shrimp can easily be swapped for the tofu. Look for tofu that has added calcium.

DRESSING

½ CUP CANOLA OIL

3 TEASPOONS SESAME OIL

¼ CUP RICE VINEGAR

3 TABLESPOONS WHEAT-FREE TAMARI

1 TABLESPOON FRESH LIME JUICE

2 TEASPOONS HONEY

2 TEASPOONS TOASTED SESAME SEEDS

2 TEASPOONS MINCED GINGER

1 GARLIC CLOVE, MINCED

KOSHER SALT AND FRESHLY GROUND BLACK PEPPER

SLAW

1 SMALL HEAD NAPA OR SAVOY CABBAGE (ABOUT 1½ POUNDS), CORED AND SHREDDED

1 POUND FIRM TOFU, CUT INTO ½-INCH CUBES

½ CUP LOOSELY PACKED FRESH BASIL

3 OUNCES MUNG BEAN SPROUTS OR SUNFLOWER SEED SPROUTS

continued ▶

10 SNOW PEAS, TRIMMED AND CUT LENGTHWISE INTO THIN STRIPS

4 SCALLIONS, SLICED ¼-INCH THICK

1 CARROT, PEELED AND CUT INTO MATCHSTICKS

1 CUCUMBER, PEELED, SEEDED, AND SLICED ¼-INCH THICK

1 THAI CHILE, SEEDED AND THINLY SLICED

½ CUP SLICED ALMONDS, TOASTED

¼ CUP TOASTED SESAME SEEDS

To make the dressing:

Combine all the ingredients in the order listed in a jar, cover, and shake vigorously.

To make the slaw:

1. Combine all the ingredients in the order listed in a large bowl. Toss to combine.

2. Serve the slaw with the dressing on the side.

Spinach Salad with Toasted Walnuts and Walnut Oil Dressing

SERVES 4

▶ CALORIES 433, FAT 42 G, CHOLESTEROL 23.6 MG, SODIUM 659 MG, CARBOHYDRATES 5.2 G, FIBER 2.6 G, PROTEIN 13 G, IRON 14.4%, FOLIC ACID 21.5%

To make this rich salad vegetarian or to boost its folic acid values, swap the pancetta for diced avocado. To make this an entrée salad, add 4 ounces of protein, such as cooked lentils or salmon, and serve with crusty whole-grain bread. The vitamin C in the orange juice aids in the absorption of iron from the spinach.

¼ CUP DICED PANCETTA OR BACON
2 TABLESPOONS ORANGE JUICE
¼ CUP WALNUT OIL
PINCH OF SALT
PINCH OF FRESHLY GROUND BLACK PEPPER
ONE 5-OUNCE PACKAGE BABY SPINACH
ONE 5-OUNCE PACKAGE MIXED BABY GREENS (SUCH AS SPRING MIX)
¼ CUP WALNUTS PIECES, TOASTED
CRUMBLED FETA OR PARMESAN FOR SERVING

1. Heat a small skillet over medium heat. Add diced pancetta and cook until the pancetta is crisp and lightly browned, about 5 minutes. Remove from the pan and set aside.

2. In a large bowl, whisk together the orange juice and walnut oil until emulsified. Whisk in the salt and pepper.

3. Wash and dry the spinach and baby greens, and toss with the dressing.

4. Sprinkle the salad with the pancetta, walnuts, and cheese. Toss gently and serve.

Rice and Lentil Salad

▶ CALORIES 477, FAT 16.5 G, CHOLESTEROL 0 MG, SODIUM 211 MG, CARBOHYDRATES 68.6 G, FIBER 12.5 G, PROTEIN 13.9 G, IRON 22.4%, FOLIC ACID 46.2%

Lentils are an outstanding source of iron and folic acid. Lentils contain 180 micrograms of folic acid in every ½-cup serving, or almost 50 percent of the recommended daily allowance. Pretty impressive! If you already have leftover cooked rice on hand, this recipe comes together in a jiffy.

2 TABLESPOONS EXTRA-VIRGIN OLIVE OIL

2 TABLESPOONS SHERRY VINEGAR OR RED WINE VINEGAR

1 TABLESPOON FINELY CHOPPED SHALLOT

1 TABLESPOON DIJON MUSTARD

½ TEASPOON PAPRIKA, PREFERABLY SMOKED

¼ TEASPOON SALT

¼ TEASPOON FRESHLY GROUND BLACK PEPPER

2 CUPS COOKED BROWN RICE

1⅓ CUPS COOKED LENTILS OR ONE 15-OUNCE CAN LENTILS, RINSED AND DRAINED

1 CARROT, PEELED AND DICED

2 TABLESPOONS CHOPPED FRESH PARSLEY

1. Whisk together the oil, vinegar, shallot, mustard, paprika, salt, and pepper in a large bowl.

2. Add the rice, lentils, carrot, and parsley. Stir to combine and serve.

Cannellini Bean Salad with Mint and Parsley

SERVES 4

▶ CALORIES 302.7, FAT 14.1 G, CHOLESTEROL 0.9 MG, SODIUM 558 MG, CARBOHYDRATES 37 G, FIBER 11.7 G, PROTEIN 13.9 G, IRON 30.4%, FOLIC ACID 1.5%

Any white or heirloom white bean works in this recipe. Feel free to change the herbs with the seasons.

TWO 15-OUNCE CANS CANNELLINI OR OTHER CANNED BEANS,
  OR HOME-COOKED WHITE BEANS
¼ CUP EXTRA-VIRGIN OLIVE OIL
¼ CUP CHOPPED FRESH MINT
¼ CUP CHOPPED FRESH PARSLEY
¼ TEASPOON SALT
1 ANCHOVY, MINCED (OPTIONAL)
1 GARLIC CLOVE, MINCED (OPTIONAL)

1. Drain and rinse the beans. In a medium bowl, combine the olive oil, mint, parsley, and salt. Add the anchovy and garlic, if using.

2. Fold the beans into the dressing and serve.

Cream of Tomato Soup

SERVES 6

▶ CALORIES 239, FAT 14 G, CHOLESTEROL 24 MG, SODIUM 316 MG, CARBOHYDRATES 26.3 G, FIBER .4 G, PROTEIN 1.8 G, IRON 9%, FOLIC ACID 1.4%

Yes, while following the fertility diet, you can eat cream again. With a bowl full of this comfort food, you'll meet the day's requirement for full-fat dairy. To peel the tomatoes, use a serrated tomato peeler or plunge the tomatoes in a pot of boiling water for 1 minute and then slip the skins off. If you do not have time to do this step, substitute two 28-ounce cans of whole peeled tomatoes and their juice.

3 TABLESPOONS EXTRA-VIRGIN OLIVE OIL

1½ CUPS CHOPPED ONIONS

1 SMALL FENNEL BULB, TRIMMED AND CHOPPED, FRONDS RESERVED

1 TABLESPOON MINCED GARLIC

4 POUNDS RIPE TOMATOES, PEELED AND COARSELY CHOPPED

1 TABLESPOON TOMATO PASTE

3 CUPS VEGETABLE STOCK

1 TEASPOON SEA SALT

2 TEASPOONS FRESHLY GROUND BLACK PEPPER

¾ CUP HEAVY CREAM

1. Heat the olive oil over medium heat in a large heavy saucepan. Add the onions and fennel and sauté for about 10 minutes, until tender. Add the garlic and cook until soft, about 1 minute.

2. Add the tomatoes, tomato paste, vegetable stock, salt, and pepper, and stir. Bring the soup to a boil, lower the heat, and simmer, uncovered, for about 30 minutes, or until the tomatoes are tender.

3. Whisk the cream into the soup and warm over low heat just until hot. Garnish with the reserved fennel fronds and serve.

Tomato Bean Soup with Farro

SERVES 8

▶ CALORIES 126, FAT 3.9 G, CHOLESTEROL 0 MG, SODIUM 185.7 MG, CARBOHYDRATES 21 G, FIBER 3 G, PROTEIN 3.9 G, IRON 8.7%, FOLIC ACID 6.7%

This soup is a quick and inexpensive introduction to farro, an ancient form of wheat. It is easier to digest than modern wheat because it has less gluten, and it is digested more slowly, which helps keep blood sugar levels stable. You'll find traditional Italian farro or German emmer wheat, a good substitute, at a health food store or specialty foods store. If you cannot find either one, substitute bulgur.

2 TABLESPOONS EXTRA-VIRGIN OLIVE OIL
1 MEDIUM ONION, DICED
1 CELERY STALK, DICED
2 GARLIC CLOVES, MINCED
8 CUPS VEGETABLE BROTH OR WATER
1 CUP DRIED WHITE BEANS, SOAKED OVERNIGHT, RINSED, AND DRAINED
ONE 14-OUNCE CAN DICED TOMATOES, WITH THEIR JUICE
1 CUP FARRO OR EMMER
½ TEASPOON DRIED THYME
2 BAY LEAVES
½ TEASPOON FRESHLY GROUND BLACK PEPPER
SEA SALT

1. Heat the olive oil in a large soup pot over medium-high heat. Add the onion, celery, and garlic, and sauté until tender, about 8 minutes.

2. Add the broth, beans, tomatoes, farro, thyme, bay leaves, and pepper, and bring to a simmer.

3. Lower the heat, cover, and simmer for 2 hours, or until the beans and farro are tender.

4. Season with sea salt and more freshly ground pepper to taste.

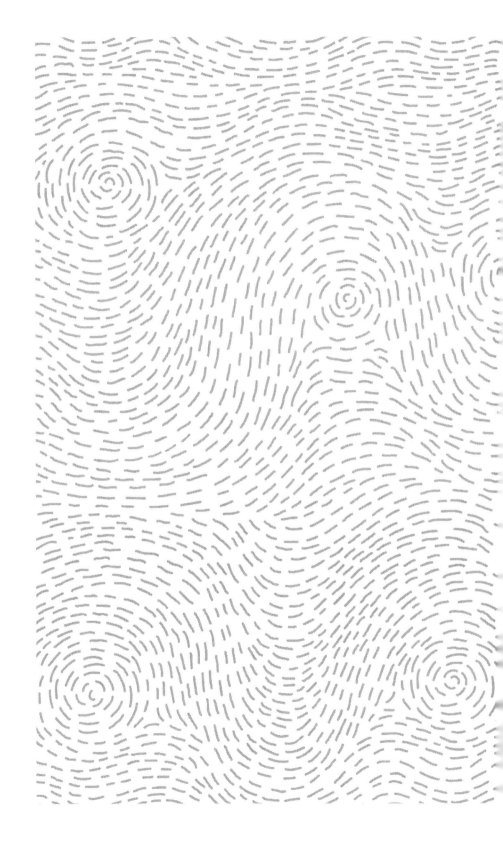

Dinner

Buffalo Burgers with Smoky Flavors

SERVES 4

▶ CALORIES 267, FAT 6 G, CHOLESTEROL 85 MG, SODIUM 326 MG, CARBOHYDRATES 16 G, FIBER .5 G, PROTEIN 35 G, IRON 14.4%, FOLIC ACID 4.9%

Buffalo is a lean red meat, raised from start to finish on grass. It is never fed corn or by-products, so its meat has a clean, fresh flavor. Because it is low in fat, it cooks more quickly than conventional beef burgers.

1 POUND GROUND BUFFALO (AMERICAN BISON) MEAT
¼ CUP COOKED WHOLE-GRAIN BROWN AND WILD RICE BLEND, SUCH AS LUNDBERG'S
1 TEASPOON CRACKED BLACK PEPPER
1 TEASPOON CHIPOTLE CHILE POWDER
1 TEASPOON SEA SALT
½ ONION, MINCED
2 OUNCES SMOKED GOUDA CHEESE, CUT INTO ¼-INCH CUBES
¼ CUP CHIPOTLE BARBECUE SAUCE, PLUS EXTRA FOR SERVING
SPELT BREAD FOR SERVING

1. Build a medium fire in a charcoal grill or heat a gas grill to medium.

2. In a large bowl, combine the buffalo, rice, pepper, chile powder, salt, onion, and barbecue sauce until well mixed. Shape into 4 patties.

3. Place patties on the grill and cook for about 3 minutes on each side. Serve on the spelt bread, topped with extra barbecue sauce.

Citrus-Soy Salmon

SERVES 4

▶ CALORIES 336, FAT 12.8 G, CHOLESTEROL 85 MG, SODIUM 378 MG, CARBOHYDRATES 5.7 G, FIBER 0 G, PROTEIN 47 G, IRON 6.9%, FOLIC ACID 4%

Lime juice and soy sauce are a tasty combination that complements the salmon. A bit of honey adds a nice caramel note when the fish is broiled. Substitute Arctic char when salmon is out of season. This dish is delicious served with Coconut Ginger Rice (page 83). Use any leftover salmon in a sandwich or to top a salad.

MARINADE

2 TABLESPOONS FRESH LIME JUICE

2 TABLESPOONS LOW-SODIUM SOY SAUCE

1 TEASPOON HONEY

FOUR 6-OUNCE SALMON FILLETS

SAUCE

½ CUP VEGETABLE STOCK

2 TABLESPOONS MIRIN

½ TEASPOON SALT

Preheat the broiler and oil the rack of a broiler pan.

To marinate the salmon:

In a large shallow dish, such as a pie plate, stir together the lime juice, soy sauce, and honey. Add the fish, skin-side up, cover with plastic wrap, and marinate at room temperature for 10 minutes.

To make the sauce:

1. Combine the vegetable stock, mirin, and salt in a small saucepan and boil until thickened, stirring frequently, about 4 minutes. Remove from the heat.

2. Place the fish on the rack in the broiling pan, skin-side down. Broil 5 to 7 inches from the heat until just cooked through, about 6 minutes. Spoon the sauce over the fish and serve.

Coconut Ginger Rice

SERVES 4

▶ CALORIES 370, FAT 17.8 G, CHOLESTEROL 0 MG, SODIUM 21.7 MG, CARBOHYDRATES 48 G, FIBER 3.6 G, PROTEIN 5.5 G, IRON 6.2%, FOLIC ACID 2%

Ginger promotes good blood circulation, and during pregnancy, it also helps alleviate nausea. Coconut oil is a saturated fat, but recent research indicates that the fat in virgin coconut oil is composed mainly of medium-chain tri-glycerides, which may not carry the same risks as other saturated fats. Look for coconut oil and coconut milk in Asian markets, health food stores, and well-stocked grocery stores.

2 TABLESPOONS VIRGIN COCONUT OIL

1 TABLESPOON MINCED FRESH GINGER

1½ CUPS WHOLE-GRAIN BROWN AND WILD RICE BLEND,
    SUCH AS LUNDBERG'S

3 CUPS FILTERED WATER

ONE 5-OUNCE CAN (ABOUT ½ CUP) UNSWEETENED COCONUT MILK

½ TEASPOON SALT

1 BAY LEAF

2 TABLESPOONS CHOPPED SCALLION

1. In a medium saucepan, heat the coconut oil over medium-high heat until hot, but not smoking. Add the ginger and sauté for 2 minutes. Add the water, coconut milk, salt, and bay leaf, and bring to a boil.

2. Reduce the heat to low and cook, covered, for 20 minutes, or until the liquid is absorbed.

3. Remove the pan from the heat and sprinkle with the scallions. Let stand for 5 minutes. Remove the bay leaf, fluff with a fork, and serve.

Yellow Dal with Split Peas

SERVES 4

▶ CALORIES 187, FAT .5 G, CHOLESTEROL 0 MG, SODIUM 253.7 MG, CARBOHYDRATES 32.6 G, FIBER 11.4 G, PROTEIN 11.9 G, IRON 17.6%, FOLIC ACID 16%

Dal is a staple of Indian cuisine. This dish gets a burst of color and an aromatic flavor from the turmeric. The cayenne can really pack some heat, so taste the dal before adding more. Serve it with a green salad and wild rice.

1 CUP YELLOW SPLIT PEAS OR MOONG DAL

2 CUPS WATER OR VEGETABLE BROTH

1 TEASPOON GROUND TURMERIC

¼ TEASPOON CAYENNE PEPPER

½ TEASPOON SALT

1 TABLESPOON MARGARINE

1 ONION, CHOPPED

1½ TEASPOONS GROUND CUMIN

2 WHOLE CLOVES

1 BUNCH BROCCOLI RABE (ABOUT ½ POUND), TRIMMED, STEAMED, AND CUT INTO 1-INCH PIECES

1. In a large pot, combine the split peas and water and bring to a slow simmer. Add the turmeric, cayenne, and salt, and cover. Cook for about 20 minutes, stirring occasionally.

2. In a medium skillet, melt the margarine over medium-high heat. Add the onion, cumin, and cloves. Sauté for 4 to 6 minutes, or until the onion is soft. Add the onion mixture to the split peas and stir.

3. Simmer the dal for 5 minutes, or until the lentils are tender. Remove the cloves, stir in the broccoli rabe, and serve.

Roasted Balsamic Brussels Sprouts with Pignoli

SERVES 4

▶ CALORIES 131, FAT 12.1 G, CHOLESTEROL 0 MG, SODIUM 11 MG, CARBOHYDRATES 3.6 G, FIBER, 1.9 G, PROTEIN 2.7 G, IRON 3.4%, FOLIC ACID 6.7%

This is a terrific recipe for those who think they don't like Brussels sprouts, because roasting them brings out their sweetness. Any nut works here, and you can also toss in a cooked and diced bacon strip.

20 TO 25 MEDIUM BRUSSELS SPROUTS (ABOUT 1 POUND), HALVED
2 TABLESPOONS EXTRA-VIRGIN OLIVE OIL
SEA SALT
FRESHLY GROUND BLACK PEPPER
¼ CUP CHOPPED PIGNOLI NUTS, TOASTED
1 TABLESPOON BALSAMIC VINEGAR

1. Preheat the oven to 400°F.

2. Spread out the Brussels sprouts in a single layer on a baking sheet. Drizzle with the olive oil, and sprinkle with the sea salt and pepper.

3. Roast for 20 to 25 minutes, or until the Brussels sprouts are tender and caramelized.

4. Remove from the oven and sprinkle with the pignoli nuts.

5. Toss with the vinegar and serve.

Old-Fashioned Stuffed Peppers

SERVES 6

▶ CALORIES 234.7, FAT 7 G, CHOLESTEROL 33.6 MG, SODIUM 434 MG, CARBOHYDRATES 11.4 G, FIBER 1 G, PROTEIN 9.5 G, IRON 2.3%, FOLIC ACID 4.8%

Red bell peppers have more nutrients than green or yellow ones, including plenty of vitamin C and carotenoids. The yogurt and feta cheese give this dish a Greek twist.

6 RED BELL PEPPERS
¾ CUP WHOLE-MILK FETA CHEESE
¾ CUP COOKED WHOLE-GRAIN BROWN AND WILD RICE BLEND,
    SUCH AS LUNDBERG'S
½ CUP PLAIN UNSWEETENED GREEK YOGURT
¼ CUP MINCED ONION
¼ CUP EXTRA-VIRGIN OLIVE OIL
1 TEASPOON DRIED OREGANO
½ TEASPOON DRIED DILL WEED
½ CUP TOMATO SAUCE OR JUICE

1. Preheat the oven to 350°F.

2. Cut the tops off the peppers and set aside. Core and seed the peppers.

3. Combine the cheese, rice, yogurt, onion, olive oil, oregano, and dill in a food processor. Pulse for 30 seconds, or until just blended.

4. Carefully spoon the stuffing into the peppers. Put the tops back on the peppers.

5. Place the stuffed peppers in a 9-inch square pan and pour the tomato sauce in. Cover with aluminum foil and bake for 30 minutes. Remove the foil and bake for 30 minutes, or until the peppers are cooked through and the tops are lightly charred and beginning to wrinkle.

Salmon Poke

SERVES 4 AS AN APPETIZER OR 2 AS A MAIN COURSE

▶ CALORIES 277.7, FAT 15.2 G, CHOLESTEROL 64.6 MG, SODIUM 635.7 MG, CARBOHYDRATES 1.4 G, FIBER .6 G, PROTEIN 32.4 G, IRON 8.9%, FOLIC ACID 3.9%

Poke is a Hawaiian dish made with raw fish. This one includes the crisped skin, which adds great texture and is a terrific, often overlooked source of omega-3 fatty acids.

ONE 8-OUNCE FILLET OF SUSHI-GRADE ALASKAN SOCKEYE SALMON, SKIN REMOVED AND RESERVED (THE FISHMONGER CAN REMOVE IT)
2 TEASPOONS WHEAT-FREE TAMARI
2 TEASPOONS SESAME OIL
1 TABLESPOON TOASTED SESAME SEEDS
1 SHEET NORI, SHREDDED BY HAND OR WITH SCISSORS

1. Preheat the oven to 350°F.

2. Cut the salmon into ½-inch dice and put into a large mixing bowl.

3. Line a baking sheet with foil or parchment paper and spread out the skin so the fleshy side is up. Bake until crispy, about 20 minutes. Cool, cut into thin strips, and set aside.

4. Drizzle the salmon with tamari and sesame oil, and toss to combine.

5. Sprinkle with the sesame seeds, nori, and crispy salmon skin, and serve.

Mackerel and Lentil Salad

SERVES 4

▶ CALORIES 533.9, FAT 41.9 G, CHOLESTEROL 88.6 MG, SODIUM 400.1 MG, CARBOHYDRATES 9.9 G, FIBER 1.8 G, PROTEIN 30 G, IRON 12.5.9%, FOLIC ACID 4.7%

This main-dish salad packs a double-dose of oily fish. If you are just dipping your toes into the world of oil-rich fish, you can tone down the strength of the fish flavors by leaving out either the mackerel or the anchovies.

2 TABLESPOONS CANOLA OIL

1 CELERY STALK, DICED

2 CARROTS, PEELED AND DICED

2 SMALL ONIONS, ONE CHOPPED AND THE OTHER THINLY SLICED
    LENGTHWISE

2 GARLIC CLOVES, MINCED

1 CUP LENTILS, ANY COLOR

KOSHER SALT

1½ CUPS WATER OR CHICKEN STOCK

4 OUNCES SMOKED ATLANTIC MACKEREL, SMOKED TROUT,
    OR SMOKED HERRING

2 ANCHOVY FILLETS, CHOPPED

JUICE OF 1 LEMON

¼ CUP CHOPPED FRESH PARSLEY

¼ CUP EXTRA-VIRGIN OLIVE OIL

1. In a medium sauté pan, heat the canola oil over medium heat until shimmering. Add the celery, carrots, the chopped onion, and garlic, and sauté until the vegetables are softened and beginning to caramelize, about 8 minutes.

2. Add the lentils, sprinkle with salt, and add the water. Stir to combine. Bring to a low boil, lower the heat, and simmer uncovered, until the lentils are cooked but still a bit firm to the bite, about 20 minutes. Add water ¼ cup at a time, if needed during cooking, to prevent scorching. Remove from the heat.

3. Transfer the lentils to a large, heat-proof serving bowl. Remove the skin from the mackerel and flake the fish. Distribute on top of the lentils.

4. Add the sliced onion, anchovies, lemon juice, and parsley. Add the olive oil, stir to combine, and serve.

Grilled Bluefish

SERVES 4

▶ CALORIES 588.7, FAT 57.3 G, CHOLESTEROL 89 MG, SODIUM 300 MG, CARBOHYDRATES 1 G, FIBER .2 G, PROTEIN 30 G, IRON 5.9%, FOLIC ACID 4.7%

The citrus in this dish gives it a bright, tropical flavor. If you can find small whole bluefish, grill them whole. Otherwise, fillets work fine. Bluefish is a good source of selenium and vitamins B6 and B12. Serve the fish with quinoa or couscous to soak up the sauce.

MARINADE

1 CUP EXTRA-VIRGIN OLIVE OIL

½ CUP WHITE WINE

¼ CUP FRESH BASIL LEAVES, CUT DIAGONALLY INTO ¼-INCH RIBBONS

JUICE AND ZEST OF 2 LEMONS OR ORANGES

2 TO 3 GARLIC CLOVES, MINCED

1 TEASPOON GROUND CUMIN

1 TEASPOON DRIED MARJORAM

2 PINCHES OF CAYENNE PEPPER

OLIVE OIL

4 SMALL WHOLE BLUEFISH OR FOUR 6-OUNCE BLUEFISH FILLETS

SEA SALT

FRESHLY GROUND BLACK PEPPER

1. To make the marinade: Combine all the ingredients in the order listed in a small bowl, stirring to blend.

2. Pour half the marinade into a plastic bag or a shallow dish, such as a pie plate, and add the fish. Set the remaining marinade aside to use as sauce. Refrigerate the fish, covered, for at least 1 hour.

3. Build a medium-high fire in a charcoal grill or heat a gas grill to medium-high. Brush the grate with olive oil, and grill the fish for 6 to 8 minutes, turning halfway through the cooking time.

4. Meanwhile, warm the reserved marinade. Season the fish with salt and pepper, and serve with the marinade.

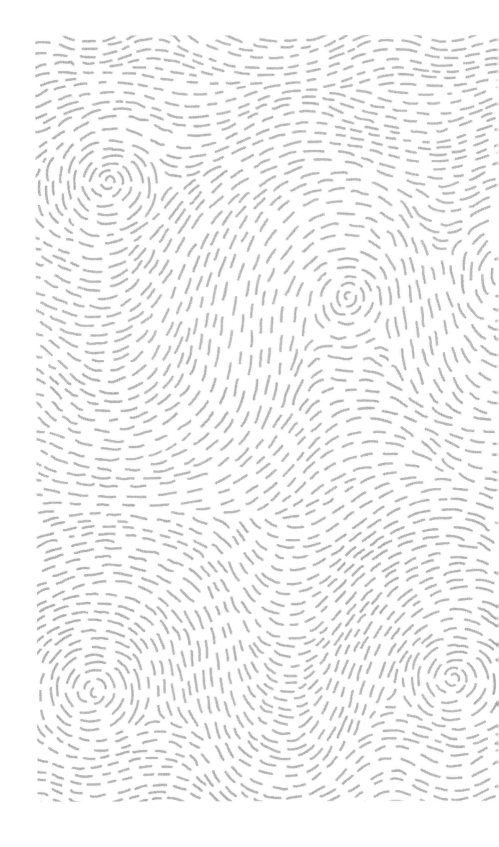

Notes

Chapter 1

Page 5: They lead to a viable pregnancy about 25 percent of the time: Chavarro, Jorge, MD, ScD; Willett, Walter, MD, DrPH, and Skerrett, Patrick J., *The Fertility Diet*, McGraw-Hill, 2009, p. 1

Page 6: This is especially true of competitive athletes who have a very low ratio of body fat to total body weight: Weschler, Toni, MPH, *Taking Charge of Your Fertility*. Harper-Collins, 2006, p. 111

Page 7: For women between 40 and 44, about 34 percent of pregnancies supposedly end in miscarriage: Twenge, Jean M., Ph.D, *The Impatient Woman's Guide to Getting Pregnant*, Atria Paperback, 2012, p. 107

Page 8: Women under 25 have a 96 percent chance of conceiving within a year: David, Sami S., MD and Blakeway, Jill, LAc, *Making Babies: A Proven 3-Month Program for Maximum Fertility*, p. 60

Page 8: One in three couples experienced a miscarriage when the man was 45 or older: Ibid., p. 61

Page 10: It will normally register somewhere between 97°F and 97.7°F: Weschler, Toni, p. 53

Page 11: On average, fertile cervical fluid lasts for three days: David and Blakeway, p. 37

Page 11: The pH level of fertile cervical fluid: David and Blakeway, p. 38

Page 12: A wider "gate" for the sperm to pass through: Weschler, p. 64

Page 16: ...remain elevated for more than eighteen days: David and Blakeway, p. 47

Page 19: A woman can get pregnant during any given cycle for about seven cycle days: http://tcoyf.com/content/FertMyths.aspx

Chapter 2

Page 21: Roughly 12 percent of fertility issues stem from weight problems: David and Blakeway, p. 65

Page 21: Lack of sleep can alter your hormonal balance: Ibid., p. 68

Page 22: While studies on caffeine and fertility are inconclusive: Ibid., 75

Page 23: The activation of the adrenal glands: David and Blakeway, p. 83. All stress information pulled from Chapter 4, pp. 83–98.

Page 27: The follicles in the ovaries turn into fluid-filled sacs known as cysts: Ibid., p. 102

Page 30: Acupuncture can increase blood flow: David and Blakeway, pp. 188–189

Page 31: There have been no studies on whether Chinese herbal medicine: Twenge, p. 17

Page 31: Chinese herbs are used to increase cervical mucus: David and Blakeway, p. 189

Page 32: His choice of underwear will have no impact: Twenge, pp. 9–10

Page 32: ...play it safe by avoiding hot tubs: Ibid., p. 10

Page 32: The combination of tight shorts: Weschler, p. 175

Page 33: Almost all lubricants, from vegetable oil to petroleum jelly: Ibid., p. 172

Page 33: Douches alter the natural pH level of the vagina: Ibid., p. 174

Page 33: It allows for the deepest penetration: Ibid., p. 173

Page 33: Being overweight, with a much higher percentage of body fat: Ibid.

Page 33: For almost everyone, up to 90 milligrams of caffeine per day is considered safe: Ibid, David and Blakeway, p. 74

Page 34: No amount of alcohol is considered safe: Ibid., p. 75

Page 34: Studies have shown that men who begin a vitamin regimen: Ibid., p. 115

Page 35: A deficiency in B1 has been linked to anovulation: Ibid., p. 117

Page 36: Iron plays a key role in DNA replication: Ibid., p. 121

Page 36: Recent research has demonstrated the importance of essential fatty acids: Ibid., p. 125

Page 37: For women who are attempting to conceive: http://water.epa.gov/scitech/swguidance/fishshellfish/outreach/advice_index.cfm

Chapter 3

Page 39: This work is done by two key hormones insulin and glucagon: Ibid., Chavarro, p. 47

Page 40: ... diminish the peaks and valleys: David and Blakeway, p. 101

Page 40: The liver then responds by releasing more glucose: Chavarro, p. 47

Page 40: ... you will look for whole-grain carbohydrates: Chavarro, p. 52–53

Page 41: A few words about wheat, the glycemic index, and high glycemic foods: Davis, William, MD, *Wheat Belly*, Rodale, Inc., 2011, p. 33

Page 42: Celiac disease, a serious digestive disorder: Chavarro, p. 129

Page 44: These fats, which are high in cholesterol: David and Blakeway, p. 104

Page 44: In a large long-term study conducted by the Harvard School of Public Health and Harvard Medical School: Ibid.

Page 46: Conversely, the more full-fat dairy products in a woman's diet: Ibid., p. 109

Page 46: The study's researchers concluded: Ibid., p. 114

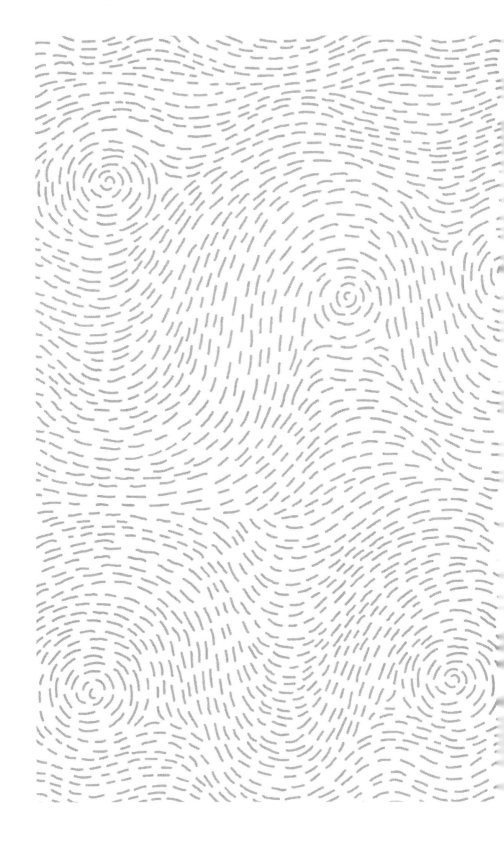

Bibliography

Chavarro, Jorge E., MD, ScD; Willett, Walter C., MD, DrPH, and Skerrett, Patrick J., *The Fertility Diet*, New York: McGraw-Hill, 2009.

David, Sami S., MD, and Blakeway, Jill, LAc, *Making Babies: A Proven 3-Month Program for Maximum Fertility*, New York: Little, Brown and Company, 2009.

Davis, William, MD, *Wheat Belly*, New York: Rodale, Inc., 2011.

Lewis, Randine, PhD, *The Infertility Cure*, New York: Little, Brown and Company, 2005.

Twenge, Jean M., PhD, *The Impatient Woman's Guide to Getting Pregnant*, New York: Free Press, 2012.

Weschler, Toni, MPH, *Taking Charge of Your Fertility*, New York: Harper Collins, 2006.

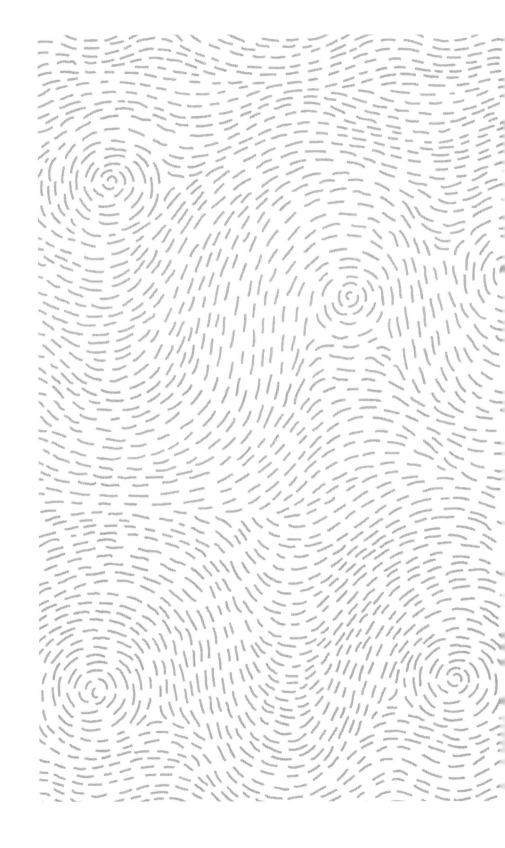

Glossary

acupuncture: The process of stimulating certain places in the body by inserting needles in the surface of the skin. In its classical form, it is a component of traditional Chinese medicine (TCM).

androgens: Male sex hormones, including testosterone. Men produce androgens in their testes, while women produce them in their ovaries and adrenal glands.

anovulation: The absence of ovulation.

anovulatory cycle: A complete menstrual cycle during which no ovulation takes place.

assisted reproductive technologies (ARTs): Methods used to achieve pregnancy by artificial or partially artificial means, such as in vitro fertilization.

basal body temperature (BBT): The lowest temperature attained by the body during rest. Taken immediately upon waking, it is also called waking body temperature.

body mass index (BMI): A number derived from a person's weight and height that provides a reliable indicator of body fatness for most people.

cervical fluid: Also called cervical mucus, it is the liquid secreted by the cervix. Semen uses cervical fluid as its mode of travel through a woman's reproductive tract.

cervix: The lower part of the uterus that projects into the vagina.

chlamydia: A prevalent, often asymptomatic, sexually transmitted disease that can lead to infertility.

circadian rhythm: The daily twenty-four-hour rhythm of biological activity and rest to which our bodies are attuned.

combined oral contraceptive pill: Referred to colloquially as the Pill, it is a birth control method that includes a combination of an estrogen (estradiol) and a progestogen (progestin). When taken by mouth every day, these pills inhibit female fertility.

conceive: To become pregnant.

conception: The process of becoming pregnant, which involves the fusion of sperm and egg.

dehydroepiandrosterone (DHEA): A precursor of male sex hormones (androgens) and female (estrogens) ones.

ectopic pregnancy: The implantation and development of a fertilized egg outside of the uterus, often in the fallopian tube.

endocrine system: A series of glands that produce chemicals called hormones.

endometriosis: A condition in which the tissue that usually lines the inside of the uterus instead grows outside of it. The misplaced tissue can appear anywhere in the abdominal cavity or within cysts in the ovaries.

endorphins: Produced by the pituitary gland and the hypothalamus during exercise, sex, and other activities, their release produces a feeling of well-being. Endorphins also increase prolactin levels.

essential fatty acids (EFAs): Fatty acids that are essential for biological processes and must be ingested from food. In humans they are alpha-linolenic acid (an omega-3 fatty acid) and linoleic acid (an omega-6 fatty acid).

estrogen: A hormone produced mainly in a woman's ovaries that is responsible for the development of secondary sex characteristics and controls the menstrual cycle.

fallopian tubes: A pair of tubes connected to the uterus. Sperm travel through the uterus to one of the fallopian tubes, where, during conception, an egg is normally fertilized. The egg travels through the tube to the uterus.

fibroids: Tumors that grown in the wall of the uterus.

follicle stimulating hormone (FSH): A hormone produced by the pituitary gland that helps the ovaries to produce mature eggs and estrogen.

follicular phase: The part of the menstrual cycle from the onset of menstruation until ovulation. Also known as preovulatory phase.

gluten: A protein composite made of a gliadin and a glutenin. Gluten is found in foods made from wheat and related grain species such as barley and rye.

glycemic index (GI): A measure of how quickly blood sugar levels rise after eating a particular type of food. The higher the blood sugar, the higher the GI.

heme iron: A form of iron sourced from animal flesh.

homeostasis: The body's ability to maintain its biochemistry by continual adjustment to the demands placed upon it, both internally and externally.

hypothalamus: A part of the brain that links the nervous system to the endocrine system via the pituitary gland.

hysterosalpingogram and hysteroscopy: Tests that use different technologies to examine the lining of the uterus and fallopian tubes to make sure there are no blockages, fibroids, or other deterrents interfering with the egg's journey to and implantation in the uterus.

in vitro fertilization (IVF): A procedure during which a woman's egg is fertilized by her partner's sperm outside of her body in a petri dish before being placed in the uterus.

insulin and glucagon: Hormones produced by the pancreas that work together to turn what you eat into a simple sugar known as glucose, which your cells use to perform their job properly.

intrauterine insemination (IUI): A procedure during which a man's sperm is injected through the cervix directly into the uterus.

libido: Sexual desire.

luteal phase: The postovulatory phase of the menstrual cycle, which lasts from ovulation until the onset of menstruation.

luteinized unruptured follicle syndrome (LUFS): When this condition is present, the egg does not get released from one of the ovary's follicles. It's believed to be a major cause of unexplained fertility.

luteinizing hormone (LH): A hormone secreted by the pituitary gland, normally released in a surge to cause ovulation.

menstrual cycle: The regular, cyclical changes in the ovaries, cervix, and lining of the uterus (endometrium) under the influence of sex hormones.

miscarriage: The spontaneous loss of the embryo or fetus from the uterus.

nonheme iron: A form of iron sourced by eating plant proteins.

ovulation: The release of a mature egg from the ovarian follicle.

ovulation predictor kit (OPK): Used to detect the impending release of an egg, usually by testing urine for the presence of the luteinizing hormone.

pelvic inflammatory disease (PID): An infection that inflames the fallopian tubes and ovaries and can cause infertility.

phytonutrient: A compound occurring naturally in plants that promotes health and helps prevent disease.

pituitary gland: A gland that produces many hormones, and influences other glands to make hormones. The pituitary hormonally controls the ovaries and testes.

polycystic ovarian syndrome (PCOS): An endocrine disorder that can cause irregular menstrual cycles and other problems. Developing follicles remain trapped in the ovary and become cysts on the internal ovarian wall. Believed to be caused by high blood insulin levels.

premature ovarian failure (POF): A condition in which a woman's ovaries stop producing eggs a decade or more before normal menopause.

premenstrual syndrome (PMS): Physical and emotional signs and symptoms that may appear during the luteal phase of the menstrual cycle.

progesterone: A hormone produced in the ovaries following ovulation. It is responsible for preparing the uterus for possible pregnancy and influences waking temperature and cervical fluid characteristics.

prolactin: A hormone produced in the pituitary gland that stimulates the production of breast milk and inhibits the production of estrogen.

pubococcygeus muscles (PCs): The muscles of the pelvic floor. They support the uterus, bladder, and rectum.

seminal ducts: A pair of sacs that open to the male's urethra, which secretes a fluid that is part of seminal fluid.

sperm: A male reproductive cell.

stress response: Also called the fight-or-flight response, it is a physiological reaction in response to an event perceived as threatening. The reaction produces a discharge from the sympathetic nervous system, which eventually results in the hormonal overproduction of adrenaline and cortisol.

testicles: A pair of male sex organs that produce sperm and androgens, including testosterone.

thyroid: An endocrine gland that manages the speed at which the body uses energy. The thyroid regulates the growth and rate of function of many other systems in the body.

traditional Chinese medicine (TCM): A range of medical practices developed in China over 2,000 years ago. Includes herbal medicine, acupuncture, massage, exercise, and dietary therapy.

uterus: The pear-shaped organ in which the fertilized egg implants and grows for the duration of pregnancy. When implantation does not occur, the lining of the uterus sheds during menstruation.

vagina: Also known as the birth canal, this muscular canal extends from the cervix to the vulva.

vulva: The external parts of a woman's genital organs—labia, clitoris, and vagina—as well as the opening to the urethra.

zygote: A fertilized egg.

Medical Terms and Acronyms

ART: Assisted reproductive technology

BBT: Basal body temperature

BMI: Body mass index

COCP: Combined oral contraceptive pill

EFA: Essential fatty acid

FSH: Follicle-stimulating hormone

GI: Glycemic index

IUI: Intrauterine insemination

IVF: In vitro fertilization

LH: Luteinizing hormone

LUFS: Luteinized unruptured follicle syndrome

ob-gyn: obstetrician/gynecologist

OPK: Ovulation predictor kit

PCs: Pubococcygeus muscles

PCOS: Polycystic ovarian syndrome

PID: Pelvic inflammatory disease

PMS: Premenstrual syndrome

POF: Premature ovarian failure

STI: Sexually transmitted infection

TCM: Traditional Chinese medicine

Resources

The Boston Women's Health Book Collective, *Our Bodies, Ourselves: A New Edition for a New Era, New York: Touchstone,* 2005. www.ourbodiesourselves.org /book/

Shettles, Landrum, M.D., Ph.D., *How to Choose the Sex of Your Baby*, New York: Broadway Books, fully revised and updated in 2006. http://Tcoyf.com/

For Current Information About Safe Seafood Choices

www.seafoodchoices.com/

http://water.epa.gov/scitech/swguidance/fishshellfish/outreach/advice_ index.cfm

http://www.montereybayaquarium.org/cr/seafoodwatch.aspx

Apps for Charting Your Fertility Signs with Your Mobile Phone

FemCal: Period and Ovulation Calendar from Dalmo Cirne

MeFertil from Watmough Software

Index

Manufactured by Amazon.ca
Bolton, ON

13734365R00063